NO-SALT COOKERY

A healthy diet, full of flavour and variety, using all the goodness of fresh, natural
ingredients.

NO-SALT COOKERY

Wholesome recipes for low-sodium eating

by

SARAH BOUNDS

Illustrated by Ian Jones
Photography by John Welburn Associates
Cookware for photography kindly loaned by Harrods

THORSONS PUBLISHERS INC.
New York

Thorsons Publishers Inc.
377 Park Avenue South
New York, New York 10016

First U.S. Edition 1984

LIBRARY OF CONGRESS CATALOGING IN PUBLICATION DATA

Bounds, Sarah
    No-salt cookery.
    Includes index.
    1. Hypertension—Diet therapy—Recipes.   2. Salt-free
    diet—Recipes.   2. Hypertension—Prevention.   I. Title.
RC685.H8B68   1984   641.5'632   84-2432
ISBN 0-7225-0896-4

Printed and bound in Great Britain

Thorsons Publishers Inc. are distributed to the trade by
Inner Traditions International Ltd., New York

CONTENTS

	Page
Introduction	7
Chapter	
1. The Salt in Our Food	11
2. Planning a Low-Salt Diet	15
3. Breakfasts	22
4. Soups and Starters	26
5. Main Courses	35
6. Vegetables and Salads	59
7. Stocks, Sauces and Dressings	69
8. Breads and Biscuits	76
9. Cakes and Desserts	83
Index	95

To Graham, for his love and support.

'I was at first at great loss for salt; but custom soon reconciled the want of it; and I am confident that the frequent use of salt among us is an effect of luxury, and was first introduced only as a provocative to drink . . . and as for myself, when I left this country, it was a great while before I could endure the taste of it in anything.'

— Jonathan Swift, *Gulliver's Travels*.

INTRODUCTION

Why Cut Down on Salt?

Wars have been fought for it; Roman soldiers were taxed on it and Gandhi marched to the sea in protest against the British policy on it. Salt has played an important part in man's life for centuries. It is essential to life. What we know as salt is actually a compound called sodium chloride. The body breaks this down to sodium and chloride, both of which are involved in maintaining the body's delicate balance of fluids. Of the two chemicals it is sodium which plays a more significant part in the body.

Sodium is found in the fluids that surround the cells of the body, where it balances the potassium present inside the cells. The presence of these two minerals enables nerve impulses to be transmitted and muscles to respond accordingly. A complex series of reactions with enzymes, called the ionic pump, ensures that the potassium stays within the cell and the sodium outside.

The two minerals help to ensure that the balance of fluids between and around cells is maintained. This is achieved through the kidneys, which regulate the availability of the minerals. If there is too much sodium the kidneys will remove the surplus, or if there is too little then the processes that remove sodium in the urine and in the sweat will be shut down.

In Britain there is little danger of sodium deficiency. We are addicted to salt. On average each of us manages to eat 12g salt a day, while research suggests that our bodies can get by with an intake of sodium as low as 200mg (from about 500mg salt). At the other end of the scale there are people who eat as much as 20g salt daily. It is easy to overdo the salt. Salt is added during cooking, at the table, and during the manufacture of many processed foods, along with other sodium-based ingredients such as monosodium glutamate or baking powder.

Now health authorities are beginning to advise a reduction in salt from the normal 12g a day to a figure around 3-5g. Back in 1977 the U.S. Senate Select Committee on Nutrition and Human Needs called for a reduction in the level of salt eaten in the American diet of between 50 and 85 per cent, to 3g a day. The Americans responded dramatically; now half the population are trying to achieve this target figure. In Britain, the Health Education Council have spelt out the dangers of too much salt in the diet and the National Advisory Committee on Nutrition Education (NACNE) has also called for a reduction in salt intake. The NACNE report, Proposals for Nutritional Guidelines for Health and Education in Britain was published last year. It recommends a reduction in salt intake and says, 'A salt intake of 12g a day is far in excess of that required even by physically active individuals and a gradual reduction to a half or even a quarter of this level is unlikely to be associated with any danger to health.'

The greatest and most widely publicised danger of too much salt in the diet is high blood pressure (hypertension). The highest level of blood pressure in the world occurs in Japan, where there is a similarly high intake of salt. At the other end of the scale there are communities where salt intake is very low, communities like the bushmen of the Kalahari desert or the Solomon islanders. One group of Solomon islanders cooks food by steaming it over water from freshwater streams. They have a low salt intake and a low incidence of high blood pressure. A second group of islanders however, eats much the same food as the first group but boils food in sea water. Their intake of salt is much higher and so is the occurrence of high blood pressure. Animal experiments have emphasized the link between salt intake and high blood pressure by inducing the latter in animals by giving them a diet very high in salt.

Researchers now believe that cutting down on salt and increasing the level of potassium can help to lower high blood pressure. Although there are no physical symptoms associated with high blood pressure, it has a significant impact on health. If you suffer from high blood pressure the chances of your experiencing a stroke, heart disease or kidney failure are all increased. It is, says Graham MacGregor of the Charing Cross Hospital's blood pressure unit, probably the most preventable cause of death in the West.

In this country between 15 and 20 per cent of all adults have high blood pressure. Blood pressure is quite simply the amount of force required to circulate the blood through the body. Blood pressure is measured by a device called a sphygmomanometer. As the heart beats the blood is forced out and along the arteries, they expand slightly to accommodate the extra volume of blood. This is the moment of highest pressure and is called the systolic pressure. This is followed by a brief pause as the pressure in the arteries falls just before the next heart beat. This is the moment of lowest pressure and is called the diastolic pressure. Normal blood pressure is usually considered to be equal to or less than a systolic level of 140mmHG and a diastolic level of, or less than, 90. High blood pressure is generally agreed to be indicated when the systolic level is at, or above, 160 and the diastolic at, or above, 95.

The level of blood pressure is constantly changing. Stress and exercise influence the level of pressure in the short term. On recovery or on resting however the level normally returns to a lower level. It is when pressure remains high and is not corrected that dangers increase.

Not everyone will develop high blood pressure. It is thought to be genetically determined; if there is family history of high blood pressure then it is likely that the individual will also develop it. But this doesn't make high blood pressure inevitable. It is now thought that by restricting the level of salt eaten, right from childhood, high blood pressure may be avoided. There are other factors which may make the development of high blood pressure more likely. Smoking, overweight and lack of exercise are all risk factors and all can be overcome with a little effort.

Cutting back on salt intake helps people with high blood pressure, because those with hypertension seem to be less able to handle salt in the body. The kidneys, which regulate sodium, are also responsible for the production of certain substances which regulate blood pressure, including renin and aldosterone. Aldosterone tends to inhibit the removal of salt and so increases the volume of blood which in turn increases pressure. Comparisons between the red blood cells of those with high blood pressure and those without have shown that, in the former, sodium and potassium were unbalanced, while in those with normal blood pressure the concentrations of the two minerals were also normal. The NACNE report concluded from calculations that reducing average salt intake to 3g a day would lead to a reduction in systolic blood pressure of 5mmHG. 'This would substantially lower the prevelance rate of hypertension and therefore the mortality resulting from the disease and associated pathology.'

Cutting down on salt intake isn't likely to have immediate effects on the blood pressure. It will take time. Blood pressure responds to salt addition or removal like an oven responds to its thermostat. Salt sets the level of pressure but does not have continuous control over it.

Restricting salt can be easy. This book is designed to help restrict the intake of salt and other sodium-rich foods by giving recipes which are full of a flavour of their own — without the need for adding salt. There are only dangers in cutting salt intake for those with special problems. Restricting salt to less than one gram a day will be dangerous for those who cannot conserve sodium in their body and who therefore need a generous regular intake. These include those suffering from Addison's disease or kidney failure. Conversely, those patients with kidney failure should not increase potassium intake. But for the rest of the population cutting down on salt and increasing potassium will do no harm and will probably do a lot of good. Those with high blood pressure and those who suffer from fluid retention will find particular benefit.

1.

THE SALT IN OUR FOOD

Salt is added to some of the most commonly eaten foods in our diet. 100g of *All Bran* contains more than 1 ½ g sodium — three times the amount we need in a whole day! A slice of bread contains about 260mg sodium, an ounce of Camembert cheese more than 300mg sodium and a rasher of bacon more than 400mg.

Salt and sodium-based additives are added to many foods, sweet and savoury. Many assume that it is the savoury foods which are responsible for our high intake of sodium, but salt and sodium-based additives are widely used to preserve, to flavour and to 'improve' many sweet foods too. Highly processed foods are usually the worst culprits as the use of additional artificial ingredients increases shelf life, flavour and texture of otherwise bland products. A careful look at the labels of processed foods is needed to keep watch on the presence of unwanted sodium-based ingredients.

In Britain, under the Food Labelling Regulations 1980, most prepacked foods must give a full list of ingredients on the label. If salt has been added to a food then it will appear as 'salt' in the ingredients list. But salt will not be declared in the ingredients list if it is part of a compound ingredient which makes up less than 25 per cent of the final food, or if the food itself is exempt from ingredient listing. This means that most processed foods, cakes, biscuits, cereals, tinned meats, tinned vegetables, fruits, fish, sauces and drinks etc., will carry a full list of ingredients. But other foods which are considered exempt from labelling requirements, such as cheese and bacon, may not reveal ingredients. Foods which aren't prepacked, or which are packed for direct sale, also need not reveal all their ingredients. Bread and cakes that are sold fresh and unwrapped are a good example.

While all bread contains salt to boost flavour, many cakes contain sodium-based baking powder to give a good rise during baking. Cakes sold prepacked in boxes or cartons will show its presence; cakes bought fresh from a baker will not.

The golden rule is to read the list of ingredients, if there is one, but you can start by reading the table on page 13 to show you which foods are high in sodium, and thus to be avoided. See the table on page 12 for a list of sodium additives which may be found in food. New labelling requirements for additives mean that some foods will be labelled with an 'E number' which refers to a specific additive. A full list of E numbers, to which additive they refer will be kept at your local library. The list below shows the E numbers for additives that are sodium-based. These should be avoided wherever possible if you are trying to cut down on sodium in your diet.

Sodium-based Additives to Avoid

E numbers are used to represent specific food additives on food labels. Here is a list of additives which are sodium-based, with their respective E number:

E201	sodium sorbate
E211	sodium benzoate
E221	sodium sulphite
E222	sodium hydrogen sulphite
E223	sodium metabisulphite
E237	sodium formate
E250	sodium nitrite
E251	sodium nitrate
E262	sodium hydrogen diacetate
E281	sodium propionate
E301	sodium-L-ascorbate
E325	sodium lactate
E331	sodium dihydrogen citrate
E331	diSodium citrate
E331	triSodium citrate
E335	sodium tartrate
E339(a)	sodium dihydrogen orthophosphate
E339(b)	diSodium hydrogen orthophosphate
E339(c)	triSodium orthophosphate
E401	sodium alginate
E450(a)	diSodium dihydrogen diphosphate
E450(a)	tetraSodium diphosphate
E450(a)	triSodium diphosphate
E450(b)	pentaSodium triphosphate
E450(c)	sodium polyphosphates
E466	carboxymethylcellulose, sodium salt
E470	sodium, potassium and calcium salts of fatty acids
E481	sodium stearoyl-2-lactylate

Other ingredients which are added to foods and contain sodium include baking powder, brine, monosodium glutamate and sodium bicarbonate.

High-sodium Foods

Bacon; ham; beefburgers; processed and preserved meats like salami, luncheon meat and corned beef; sausages, frankfurters and all bought meat pies and pasties.

Smoked fish including kippers, smoked salmon, smoked haddock etc.; all shellfish; tinned tuna fish; fishfingers and other bought fish products.

All hard cheeses; cottage cheese.

Evaporated and condensed milk.

Salted butter and margarines (not *Vitaquell, Vitaseig* or *Flora*).

Bread.

Savoury crackers and some sweet biscuits.

Many breakfast cereals including *All Bran, Weetabix*, cornflakes.

Self-raising flour.

Baked beans and all tinned vegetables (except most tinned tomatoes and Delmonte, no-salt-added range of canned vegetables).

Olives in brine.

Salted nuts, crisps and other savoury snacks.

Tomato sauce; brown sauce; Worcestershire sauce; soya sauce and miso.

Stock cubes (unless salt-free); *Marmite; Bovril; Oxo*.

Baking powder.

Foods containing sodium-based additives: monosodium glutamate; sodium benzoate; sodium bicarbonate; sodium sulphite; sodium hydroxide; sodium cyclamate; baking powder; sodium alginate; sodium propionate; bicarbonate of soda; brine.

Moderate-sodium Foods

Beef; pork; lamb; chicken; turkey; game and offal.

Fresh white and oily types of fish.

Milk (goat's milk is lower in sodium than cow's) and yogurt.

Eggs.

Cream.

Cheese, cream and curd types.

Oatmeal and cornflour.

Pulses.

Biscuits, cakes and pastries (commercial and those made with baking powder).

Some vegetables: spinach; celery; carrots; seaweed; radishes; watercress; beetroot; celeriac.

Dried fruits: apricots; currants; figs; raisins; sultanas.

White wine; brown ale and draught bitter; sherry and vermouth.

Low-sodium Foods

Brown rice.

Wholemeal flour and pasta.

Unprocessed breakfast cereals.

Unsalted butter and low-salt margarines (*Flora, Vitaquell* and *Vitaseig*).

Nuts.

Prunes.

Honey and raw cane sugars.

Fresh fruit.

Vegetables not mentioned in previous listings.

Unsalted stock cubes.

Low-sodium baking powder.

Tea and decaffeinated coffee.

Lager, pale ale and cider.

Red and rosé wines, port and spirits.

2.

PLANNING A LOW-SALT DIET

The first and most obvious step in reducing the amount of salt you eat is to cut down, or cut out altogether, the amount of salt added at table. Simply ban the salt shaker! Or take the advice of some Australian researchers who found that the amount of salt added at the table was related to the number or to the size of the salt shaker's holes! If you want to try to cut down on the amount of salt added at the table, you might seriously try blocking up some of the holes on the salt shaker.

If you are used to adding a lot of salt to the food on your plate then controlling this habit is a good starting point for restricting overall salt intake. Get into the practice of tasting the food on your plate before adding salt. After all, it's an insult to the cook to salt food automatically. The recipes in this book are all designed to be tasty enough without the need for adding extra salt, either during cooking or at the table.

There are many people, used to years of oversalting food, who will find it difficult to eat food without the accustomed taste of salt. For those who are 'addicted' to the taste, there are a number of salt replacers now available which aim to help wean people away from salt gradually. Eventually there should be no need for even a salt replacer as you will be used to enjoying your food's real flavour, unmasked by salt.

Salt replacers fall into two categories; there are low-sodium salts and salt substitutes.

Low-sodium salts: these are a half-way house, as they blend salt (sodium chloride) with other ingredients to cut down the total intake of sodium while supplying some of salt's flavour. Products include:

Cerebos Mineral Salt — a mixture of sodium chloride, potassium chloride and magnesium sulphate.

Gilbert's Biosalt — a blend of sodium chloride, phosphate, potassium bicarbonate, potassium chloride, potassium bisulphite, magnesium phosphate, iron phosphate, iron sulphate and potassium iodide.

Hofel's Sesame Salt — a mixture of ground sesame seeds and sodium chloride.

Klinge Losalt — a mixture of potassium chloride, sodium chloride and magnesium carbonate.

Prewett's *Low-sodium Salt* — a blend of sodium chloride and potassium chloride.

Salt Substitutes: these eliminate sodium chloride altogether and usually supply potassium salts in its place. Products include:

Ruthmol — a mixture of potassium chloride, lactose and edible starch.

Saltsub — a blend of potassium chloride, lactose, potassium bicarbonate, and cornflour.

Selora — a mixture of potassium chloride, potassium glutamate, glutamic acid and calcium silicate.

Trufree — potassium chloride, food starches and ammonium chloride.

American style salt substitutes are also now available in Britain. Two, *Vegit* and *Instead of Salt*, which are sold in health food shops, are based on natural herbs and spices. A British all-natural salt replacer, *Life*, is made from yeasts.

Potassium based salt substitutes perform a dual role. Free from sodium they help to control the intake of sodium in the diet and, based on potassium, they help to boost the level of this mineral in the body, which is likely to be low in those used to a high-sodium diet. Research at London's Charing Cross Hospital found potassium chloride acceptable when added to potatoes during cooking at the rate of 5g per 400g of potatoes. Above that level there was a bitter aftertaste. Many manufacturers recommend adding salt replacers or substitutes after cooking; this is an easier way to control intake. It is in the case of plainly cooked vegetables that many people feel the need to add extra salt. Alternatives to salt replacers include adding natural herbs and spices either during cooking, like adding a sprig of fresh mint to new potatoes, or serving with a well-flavoured dressing as a salad. Reducing the amount of salt used during cooking is the second step to take in cutting down on salt intake.

Replacing salt in cooking with natural flavourings ensures that food doesn't taste bland or insipid. Those used to salt will find it easier to accept well-flavoured foods. The first choice must be fresh herbs and spices for a full flavour. Parsley was once the only herb to be widely sold fresh but now more and more supermarkets are selling small packs of fresh sage, rosemary, thyme, etc. But the cheapest and easiest source of fresh herbs is home grown. It is straightforward to grow herbs yourself, either in a sunny corner of the garden or in a window-box. Alternatively, a sunny windowsill should provide enough light and warmth for even the most tricky herbs. Surplus herbs can be frozen or dried for winter use.

Prepacked herbs and spices are widely available in grocers and supermarkets. Once opened, they should be stored in air-tight containers to keep fresh longer. Experiment with different herbs and spices so you learn which flavours complement different foods and you will soon learn to appreciate more subtle flavours than that of salt!

Beware of using sodium-rich flavourings such as soya sauce, yeast extract, Worcestershire sauce etc. Look carefully at the label of compound flavouring ingredients such as these; very often they are high in salt. The *Life* range of low-sodium foods include tomato ketchup, Worcestershire sauce, brown sauce, two salad dressings, mustard and both tartare and horseradish sauce all made without the addition of salt. This is the first British range of low-sodium foods available in the UK and is sold through health food stores. Many *Health Valley* products from America are made without added sodium. These are sold in health food shops. There is also a low-sodium yeast extract, *Natex*, now available.

Choose stock cubes which are unsalted — vegetable stock cubes sold in health food stores include some salt-free varieties. The best stocks, however, are home-made. Follow the recipes for Chicken Stock (page 70), Court Bouillon (page 70) and Vegetable Stock (page 69) for successful stocks. Surplus can be frozen, for convenience, in ice cube trays. They can be used straight from the freezer as they quickly thaw out.

It is also important to watch out for sodium-based additives. As mentioned on page 11 many of the additives used in food processing are based on sodium. In the home the most likely hidden source of sodium is baking powder. Most commercial baking powders are based on sodium bicarbonate and so should be avoided. It is easy to bake cakes by alternative methods which do not depend on the addition of baking powder to give a good rise. Recipes in this book include using a rich yeast dough, a whisked sponge (where eggs and honey are whisked together to add air), folding in stiffly whisked egg whites and other techniques to give light results.

To replace conventional baking powder use either *Saltfree* baking powder (available from health food stores) or ask your chemist to make up this formula for a sodium-free baking powder:

Potassium bicarbonate	38.8g
Starch	28.0g
Tartaric acid	7.5g
Potassium bitartrate	56.1g

This should be used, suggest Charing Cross Hospital's blood pressure unit, in one and a half times the normal amount.

Just as baking cakes and biscuits at home can control the amount of sodium present so can baking bread. Salt is added to all commercially sold bread. Without salt the bread certainly tastes different; it has an almost sweet flavour. In this book you will find various bread recipes which do not contain any added salt; in its place are added natural foods which all contribute a different flavour.

Sesame and sunflower seeds, chopped walnuts, oatmeal, cracked wheat are all ingredients which add interesting flavour and texture to wholemeal bread. Simply leaving out the salt from a recipe results in a dull loaf — but you could try using only half the normal level of salt in a recipe. Mixing the dough with apple juice or natural yogurt is another way to bake a tasty loaf without the need for salt. As with any baking or cooking, it is a matter of trial and error to get the recipes right and tasting as you and your family like them. Cooking without salt is no hardship; look upon it as a challenge to be able to produce tasty dishes without the need for a grain of salt!

Eating Healthily Without Salt
This book is designed to help you cut down your salt intake while eating foods which will maintain health. The recipes are based on natural foods, foods which haven't been robbed of vital nutrients by processing and manufacturing methods. Natural foods, as well as being less likely to have had salt added, are also more nutritious than over-refined products.

Take wholemeal flour. This is produced from the whole wheat grain; nothing is added and nothing is taken away. It contains the full goodness of the wheat. White flour is produced by removing the bran and the wheatgerm. Take away the bran and you take away the valuable dietary fibre; remove the wheatgerm and vital vitamins are lost. Ensuring that the bread you eat and the flour you use are wholemeal helps to ensure that your intake of these nutrients is adequate. For the same reason choose wholemeal pasta, brown rice and other cereal products that are based on the wholegrain and are not refined.

As well as the general agreement on the importance of fibre in the diet in helping to prevent the onset of diseases as diverse as constipation and diabetes, there is a similar agreement that the levels of fat and sugar in the diet should be reduced. These recipes help to meet these demands and use predominantly vegetable oils which are high in polyunsaturated fats, thought to be beneficial in helping to prevent heart disease. The choice of fat for spreading, if you are trying to cut down on salt, lies between unsalted butter and low-salt margarines (*Flora, Vitaquell* and, for cooking, *Vitaseig*). Remember though to limit your fat intake overall.

As far as protein is concerned, it was once thought the bigger the intake the better. But nutritionists now realize there is little point in such a generous intake. Foods high in protein tend to be both expensive and high in fat. Try to limit your choice of meat to lean meat, poultry and offal; all more nutritious than fatty meats.

Meat may also contain traces of the chemicals used in rearing the animal, which in turn may build up in our bodies. It is preferable to eat fish — remembering to avoid smoked fish and shellfish because of their high salt content. Fresh fish are a healthier bet, especially oily fish like mackerel and herrings which contain a particular type of fatty acid which is beneficial in helping to protect against heart disease. Neither do fish contain traces of the poisonous chemicals to be found in meat. Free-range eggs are similarly a better buy than factory-produced eggs. The battery method of keeping chickens for laying uses chemicals to boost the hen's feed and often to colour the egg yolk. Many people feel the methods are inhumane and prefer to support less cruel methods of farming.

Plant protein foods are heavily emphasized in this book because they supply important fibre, vitamins, minerals and, with the exception of nuts, contain less fat than most animal produce. Do remember to mix different types of plant protein foods together to get adequate and balanced protein. The basic rule is to pick foods from two or more of these groups to eat at a meal — nuts and seeds, pulses (beans, peas and lentils) and grains (rice, wheat, rye, corn, millet). Alternatively, balance the protein by eating an animal protein food (meat, egg, fish, milk or cheese) with any one type of plant food. You will find the recipes in this book fulfil these basic protein combining rules to ensure that your body receives the right balance of amino acids.

Lastly, it is important to eat plenty of fresh fruit and vegetables to supply fibre and many valuable nutrients, most significantly vitamin C which is found in its richest levels in fruit and vegetables. To conserve vitamin C and the fragile B vitamins remember to cook vegetables carefully. Eat produce raw, preferably, as heat destroys both vitamins. Don't cut things up until just before they are needed, and keep cooking water to use as a base for stocks. Because vitamins B and C (and some minerals) dissolve into cooking water, many people choose to cook by steaming to retain these nutrients. Alternatively, cook in the minimum of water and save it for later use.

Fresh fruit and vegetables are doubly important in a low-salt diet because they are good sources of the mineral potassium. It is potassium, as explained previously, that is balanced in the body with sodium. Decreasing our abnormally high sodium intake is important, as is increasing our low potassium intake. Nuts, wholegrain cereals, dairy produce and fruit juices are also good sources of potassium. Ensure that your daily diet incorporates these low-sodium but high-potassium foods and you will be on the right track!

A Day's Eating Plan

Breakfast
Choose a selection of the following:

Commercial low-salt breakfast cereals such as muesli, *Shredded Wheat* or *Puffed Wheat*. Choose cereals which are made from the whole grain and which are free from added sugar.

Home-made low-salt breakfast cereal such as Breakfast Crunch (page 25) or Muesli (page 23) or porridge prepared without salt but with honey, *or* molasses, *or* dried fruit *or* sunflower seeds added for flavour instead.

Low-salt bread, Wholemeal Croissants (page 22) or Sesame and Sunflower Rolls (page 76) or Walnut Bread (page 81) served with unsalted butter or low-salt margarine and a portion of 'no-added-sugar' jam or marmalade. Alternatively limit commercial, salted wholemeal bread to four thin slices a day.

Fresh fruit added to natural yogurt, or to breakfast cereal.

Dried fruit cooked as a compote (see Cinnamon Prunes, page 23).

Free-range egg, boiled *or* poached *or* scrambled with a small amount of fat and skim milk.

Fresh fruit juice.

Lunch or Light Evening Meal
Choose from:

Sandwiches or filled rolls using bread made without salt (pages 76-82) and filled with hard-boiled eggs *or* lean meat *or* soft cheese, plus salad vegetables.

Filled, baked potato (avoiding hard cheese) and served with unsalted butter or low-salt margarine.

Large salad (see Vegetable and Salad chapter, pages 59-68).

Portion of home-made soup (see Soups and Starters, pages 26-34).

Vegetarian Scotch Egg (page 37) or Vegetable Pasty (page 40) or individual Pizza (page 38).

Dinner or Main Midday Meal
Choose a main course from pages 35-58. Alternatively grill or poach fresh fish, or choose lean meat, poultry or offal and cook without adding extra salt and with the minimum addition of fat. Serve with a suitable raw or cooked vegetable accompaniment. Follow with fresh fruit, fruit crumble, pie or any other low-salt pudding.

Drinks:

Fruit juice.

Mineral water.

Skim milk.

Goat's milk.

Yogurt-based drinks.

Herb or low-tannin teas.

Decaffeinated coffee.

Snacks:

Fresh fruit.

Raw vegetables.

Low-sodium biscuits (page 77).

Dried fruit.

Nuts, unsalted of course!

3.
BREAKFASTS

Wholemeal Croissants

(Makes 24. Each supplies 145 calories and 7mg sodium.)

Imperial (Metric)
1 oz (25g) fresh yeast
½ pint (300ml) skim milk
4 fl oz (120ml) water
1 teaspoonful honey
2 oz (50g) unsalted butter or low-salt margarine, melted and cooled
20 oz (550g) 100 per cent wholemeal flour
6 oz (175g) unsalted butter
Top of the milk to glaze

1. Crumble the yeast into a jug. Heat the milk and water until tepid and pour onto the yeast. Add the honey and the melted and cooled butter or margarine. Stir in well and leave to stand while preparing dough.

2. Rub the remaining butter into the flour until mixture resembles fine breadcrumbs.

3. Make a well in the centre of the flour and add the yeast liquid. Mix in thoroughly to form a wet dough. Cover and leave to double in size in a warm place. The mixture is now ready to use. (If liked, some can be frozen at this stage and then rolled out and baked when needed. Alternatively, the dough will keep for a couple of days, covered, in the fridge.) Divide the dough into three equal portions.

4. Roll each portion out into a circle, about 10-inches across. Cut into 8 equal segments, and roll each up into a crescent shape, starting at the widest edge, moistening the tip so that it sticks. Curl into the traditional crescent shape.

5. Transfer the crescents onto a lightly-oiled baking tray and cover. Leave to prove in a warm place until double in size. Glaze with a little top of the milk and bake in a pre-heated oven at 425°F/220°C (Gas Mark 7) for 25 minutes until golden-brown.

Muesli

(Serves 8. Supplies 330 calories and 23mg sodium per portion.)

Imperial (Metric)
3 oz (75g) dried apricots
3 oz (75g) dried dates
3 oz (75g) blanched almonds
3 oz (75g) walnuts
1½ oz (38g) sunflower seeds
12 oz (325g) rolled oats

1. Chop the apricots, dates, almonds and walnuts. Mix together with the seeds and oats.

2. The muesli is now ready to serve; moisten with a little milk, yogurt or fruit juice and, if liked, leave to soak overnight. Top with chopped fresh fruit for extra vitamin C.

Cinnamon Prunes

(Serves 4. Supplies 140 calories and 11mg sodium per portion.)

Imperial (Metric)
¾ pint (450ml) cold water
1 lemon, sliced thinly
Juice of 1 orange
2-inch piece of cinnamon
12 oz (325g) prunes

1. Put the water, lemon slices and orange juice with the cinnamon in a pan and bring to the boil.

2. Pour the liquid over the prunes so they are covered, and leave to soak overnight.

Natural Yogurt

(Makes 1 pint/600ml. Supplies 200 calories and 390mg sodium.)

Imperial (Metric)
1 pint (600ml) skim milk
1 tablespoonful skimmed milk powder
1 tablespoonful natural yogurt

1. Place the milk in a saucepan and heat to 110°F/50°C.

2. While the milk is warming, mix the yogurt and skimmed milk powder and put in the base of a wide-necked vacuum flask.

3. Pour heated milk onto starter and stir in thoroughly. Cover flask tightly and leave to incubate for 6-8 hours. Place in fridge to chill before serving.

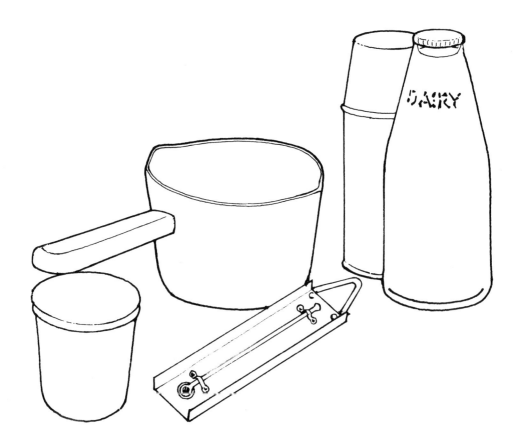

Breakfast Crunch

(Makes 2½ lb/1 kilo. Each 2 oz/50g serving supplies 220 calories and 14mg sodium.)

Imperial (Metric)
1 lb (450g) rolled oats
2 oz (50g) sesame seeds
2 oz (50g) wheatgerm
2 oz (50g) sunflower seeds
4 oz (100g) raisins
2 oz (50g) hazelnuts, chopped
2 oz (50g) almonds, blanched and chopped
2 oz (50g) desiccated coconut
¼ pint (150ml) water
¼ pint (150ml) sunflower oil
2 tablespoonsful clear honey
2 oz (50g) molasses sugar
½ teaspoonful natural vanilla essence

1. In a large mixing bowl, place the oats, seeds, wheatgerm, raisins, chopped nuts and coconut. Stir in thoroughly.

2. Bring the water to the boil and stir in the oil, honey, sugar and vanilla. Pour onto oat mixture and stir in thoroughly until well mixed.

3. Spread mixture out thinly on lightly-greased baking sheets and bake at 375°F/190°C (Gas Mark 5) for 35-40 minutes until golden-brown. Stir the mixture around halfway through cooking to make sure it bakes evenly.

4. Leave to cool and then transfer to an airtight container. Eat with skim milk or natural yogurt.

4.
SOUPS AND STARTERS

Courgette and Tarragon Soup

Illustrated opposite page 32.

(Serves 4. Supplies 80 calories and 6mg sodium per portion.)

Imperial (Metric)
2 oz (50g) onion
3 oz (75g) potato
1 tablespoonful oil
12 oz (325g) courgettes
1½ pints (900ml) vegetable stock
Sprig of fresh tarragon *or* ¼ teaspoonful dried
Freshly ground black pepper

1. Finely chop the onion and potato and sauté together, without browning, in the oil for 5 minutes.

2. While cooking, roughly chop the courgettes. Add to the pan with the stock and tarragon. Bring to the boil then cover, reduce heat and simmer for 20 minutes until vegetables are tender.

3. Remove the tarragon and liquidize soup. Return to the heat and reheat adding pepper to taste. Serve hot, if liked with swirls of natural yogurt on top of bowls.

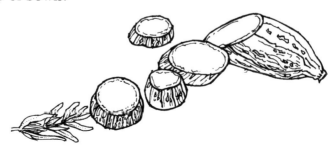

Mulligatawny Soup

Illustrated opposite page 32.

(Serves 3. Supplies 110 calories and 73mg sodium per portion.)

Imperial (Metric)
6 oz (175g) carrot
4 oz (100g) onion or leek
4 oz (100g) potato
1 green pepper
2 cloves garlic
1 dessert apple
1 tablespoonful oil
1 tablespoonful wholemeal flour
½ teaspoonful ground coriander
1 teaspoonful ground cumin
¼ teaspoonful cayenne pepper
½ teaspoonful garam masala
1½ pints (900ml) water
8 oz (225g) tomatoes (preferably fresh)
1 tablespoonful red lentils
Freshly ground black pepper

1. Dice the carrot, onion and potato. De-seed and core the pepper and chop. Crush the garlic cloves and core and chop the apple. Sauté all together in the oil for a few minutes.

2. Stir in the flour and mix well. Add the curry spices and blend well. Add the water, tomatoes and lentils. Bring to the boil, then cover, reduce heat and cook for 30 minutes.

3. Liquidize the soup and reheat, adjust seasoning to taste.

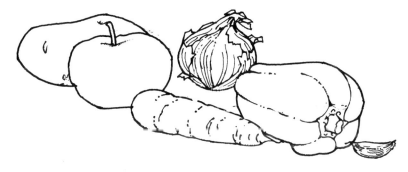

Sweetcorn Chowder

Illustrated opposite page 32.

(Serves 4. Supplies 135 calories and 49mg sodium per portion.)

Imperial (Metric)
6 oz (175g) onion
6 oz (175g) potato
1 tablespoonful oil
4 oz (100g) button mushrooms
4 oz (100g) frozen sweetcorn kernels
½ pint (300ml) skim milk
1 pint (600ml) water
1 bay leaf
½ teaspoonful thyme
Freshly ground black pepper

1. Finely chop the onion. Scrub and dice the potato. Wipe and chop the mushrooms.

2. Cook onion and potato in oil over a low heat for 3 minutes. Stir in the mushrooms, sweetcorn, milk, water and herbs. Bring to the boil then reduce heat, cover and simmer for 20 minutes.

3. Remove bay leaf. Liquidize soup reserving 2 tablespoonsful of mixture to give the soup texture. Reheat soup and season· with pepper.

Cauliflower Soup

(Serves 4. Supplies 100 calories and 3.5mg sodium per portion.)

Imperial (Metric)
1 small cauliflower
4 oz (100g) onion
4 oz (100g) potato
1 tablespoonful oil
1¼ pints (750ml) water
2 bay leaves
Pinch of rosemary
¼ pint (150ml) skim milk
Freshly ground black pepper
Chives *or* parsley, to garnish

1. Break the cauliflower into florets. Finely chop the onion and peel and dice the potato. Cook all together in the oil for a few minutes.

2. Add water and herbs plus milk. Bring to the boil, cover, reduce heat and simmer for 30 minutes.

3. Remove the bay leaves. Liquidize soup. Reheat, season with black pepper to taste and serve garnished with chopped chives or parsley.

Minestrone

(Serves 4. Supplies 120 calories and 35mg sodium per portion.)

Imperial (Metric)
1 large onion
4 oz (100g) carrot
4 oz (100g) potato
4 oz (100g) white cabbage
1 clove garlic
1 dessertspoonful oil
8 oz (225g) fresh tomatoes, skinned and chopped
½ teaspoonful oregano
2 bay leaves
2 pints (1.2 litres) water
2 oz (50g) wholemeal pasta rings
Freshly ground black pepper

1. Finely chop the onion. Scrub the carrot and potato and dice finely. Thinly shred the cabbage and crush the garlic.

2. Heat the oil and sauté all the vegetables together for 2 minutes.

3. Add the tomatoes, oregano, bay leaves and water. Bring to the boil then cover, reduce heat and simmer for 30 minutes.

4. Add pasta and cook for a further 12 minutes until pasta is just soft. Season with freshly ground black pepper and serve.

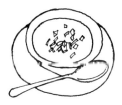

Mushrooms à la Grecque

(Serves 2. Supplies 170 calories and 12mg sodium per portion.)

Imperial (Metric)
8 oz (225g) button mushrooms
2 cloves garlic
2 ripe tomatoes
2 tablespoonsful olive oil
1 tablespoonful dry cider
1 tablespoonful salt-free tomato purée
4 fl oz (120ml) cold water
4 coriander seeds
1 bay leaf
Pinch of dried thyme *or* sprig of fresh
Pinch of dried oregano *or* sprig of fresh
Freshly ground black pepper

1. Wipe the mushrooms to remove any dirt.

2. Crush the garlic and skin and finely chop the tomatoes. Place the garlic and tomatoes in a pan with the remaining ingredients (not the mushrooms) and bring to the boil. Cook gently for 5 minutes.

3. Add the mushrooms to the pan and cook gently for 5 minutes until the mushrooms are just soft, but not soggy. Gently lift out with a slotted spoon and place in two serving dishes.

4. Cook the sauce over a fierce heat for 5 minutes to reduce it. Rub through a sieve and pour over the mushrooms. Leave to cool and serve cold.

Stuffed Tomatoes

(Serves 4. Supplies 130 calories and 6mg sodium per portion.)

Imperial (Metric)
4 large tomatoes
2 oz (50g) long-grain brown rice
1 small onion
Smear of olive oil
2 oz (50g) button mushrooms
1 oz (25g) almond slivers
1 tablespoonful chopped parsley
Freshly ground black pepper

1. Cut a thin slice from the top of each tomato. Carefully scoop out the centres and discard the seeds. Chop the flesh.

2. Place the rice in a pan of cold water. Bring to the boil, cover and reduce heat to a simmer. Cook for 25-35 minutes until just soft. Drain and set aside to cool.

3. While the rice is cooking, finely chop the onion and mushrooms. Cook the onion in the oil for a few minutes over a low heat, to soften without browning. Add the mushrooms and cook for a further 2 minutes. Heat the oven to 400°F/200°C (Gas Mark 6).

4. Remove from the heat and stir in the chopped tomato flesh, almond slivers, cooked rice and parsley. Season with pepper and pile into the 4 tomato shells. Arrange in a heatproof dish and bake for 20 minutes. Serve hot.

Celery, Apple and Walnut Starter

(Serves 4. Supplies 190 calories and 40mg sodium per portion.)

Imperial (Metric)
4 sticks celery
2 oz (50g) walnuts
2 oz (50g) raisins
2 red skinned apples
Juice of ½ a lemon
1 tablespoonful mayonnaise
1 tablespoonful natural yogurt
Freshly ground black pepper

1. Finely chop the celery. Chop the walnuts. Mix together with the raisins and celery.

2. Cut the apples into quarters and remove the core. Dice finely and mix with the lemon juice to prevent browning. Add to the other vegetables and toss in the mayonnaise and yogurt. Season with pepper.

3. Mix the ingredients together thoroughly and pile onto beds of lettuce leaves arranged in small sundae glasses.

Stuffed Courgettes

(Serves 4 as a starter. Supplies 90 calories and 6mg sodium per portion.)

Imperial (Metric)
4 small courgettes or 2 large
2 oz (50g) onions
1 dessertspoonful vegetable oil
2 oz (50g) mushrooms
½ teaspoonful dried basil *or* sprig of fresh, chopped
1 tablespoonful salt-free tomato purée
2 oz (50g) long-grain brown rice, cooked
1 dessertspoonful water
Freshly ground black pepper
2 tablespoonsful cold water

1. Cut the courgettes in half lengthwise. Using a teaspoon carefully scoop out the centre leaving ¼-inch (5mm) all round. Finely chop the flesh and set the skins aside.

2. Finely chop the onion and cook gently in the oil, without browning, for 2 minutes. Finely chop the mushrooms and add to the pan with the chopped courgette flesh. Cook gently for 2 minutes then stir in the basil, tomato and cooked rice and water. Cook gently together for a further 2 minutes then season to taste with black pepper.

3. Place the courgette skins in a shallow ovenproof dish. Divide the filling between the four and press in well. Pour the water into the dish to prevent the shells from sticking and cover with foil. Place in a pre-heated oven at 400°F/200°C (Gas Mark 6) for 15 minutes. Serve hot.

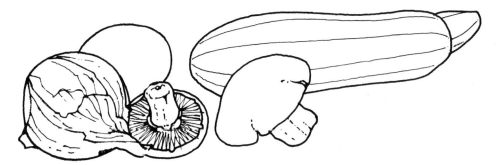

Opposite: Winter warmers. From the top: Mulligatawny Soup (page 27); Courgette and Tarragon Soup (page 26); Sweetcorn Chowder (page 28).

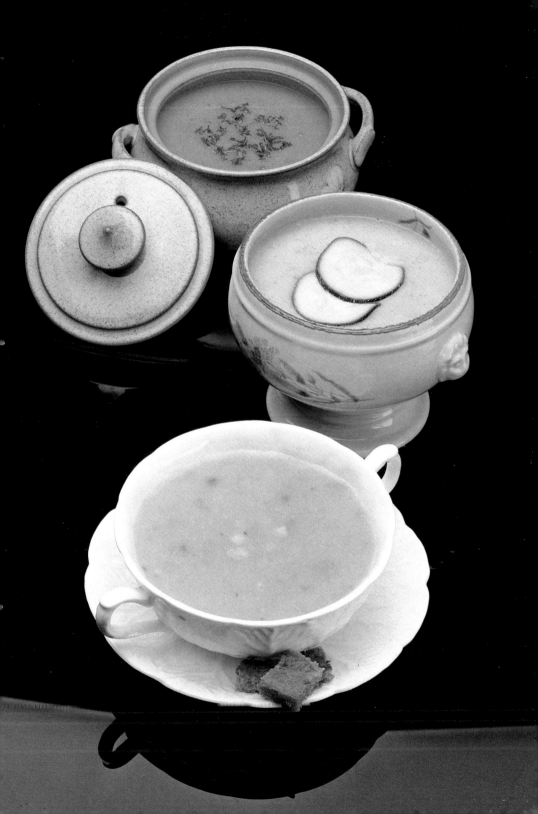

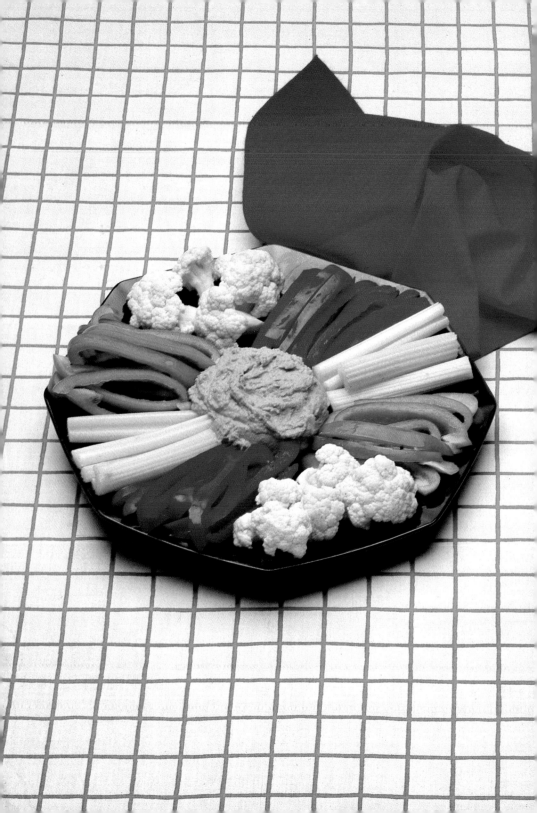

Hummus

Illustrated opposite.

(Serves 4 as a dip for crudités. Supplies 180 calories and 20mg sodium.)

Imperial (Metric)
4 oz (100g) chick peas, soaked overnight
2 cloves garlic
3 tablespoonsful tahini
Pinch paprika
½ teaspoonful ground cumin
2 tablespoonsful cold water
Juice of ½ a lemon
Freshly ground black pepper

1. Cook chick peas until soft. This is quickest in a pressure cooker; they need only 15 minutes at 15 lb (6 kilos) pressure.

2. Finely chop the garlic. When the chick peas are cooked, put in a liquidizer with the remaining ingredients and blend until smooth. Pile onto dish and chill until required.

3. Serve as a dip with crudités (strips of raw vegetables); choose from celery, green or red peppers, cucumber, carrot, courgette or cauliflower florets.

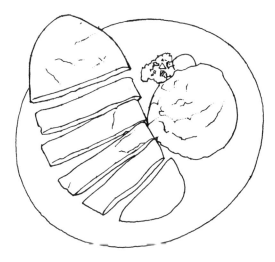

Opposite: A perfect starter. Hummus served with Crudités (above).

Guacamole

(Serve as a dip with crudités. Supplies 500 calories and 15mg sodium in total.)

Imperial (Metric)
2 ripe avocado pears
1 tablespoonful chopped onion
2 fresh tomatoes
1 fresh green chilli
2 cloves garlic
1 teaspoonful fresh lemon juice
Freshly ground black pepper

1. Remove the stones from the avocados and chop the flesh. Place in a liquidizer with the chopped onion.

2. Skin the tomatoes and discard the seeds. Put the flesh in the liquidizer.

3. De-seed and finely chop the chilli and crush the garlic. Add to the liquidizer with the lemon juice and pepper.

4. Blend until almost smooth. Turn the mixture out into a small bowl and serve with strips of prepared vegetables — carrots; cucumber; courgette; celery; cauliflower florets.

5.
MAIN COURSES

Mackerel Parcels

(Serves 4. Supplies 160 calories and 75mg sodium per portion.)

Imperial (Metric)
4 small mackerel (about 8 oz/225g each)
Juice of a lemon
Freshly ground black pepper
1 small onion
½ oz (13g) unsalted butter
4 oz (100g) button mushrooms
2 tablespoonsful chopped parsley

1. Clean the fish (or ask the fishmonger to do this). Wash and wipe dry.

2. Rub the insides of the fish with lemon juice and season with freshly ground black pepper.

3. Finely chop the onion and cook gently in the butter without browning.

4. Wipe and finely chop the mushrooms and add to the onion mixture. Cook for one minute. Remove from heat and stir in the parsley.

5. Divide the stuffing between the four fish. Place inside the fish.

6. Wrap each fish in a piece of foil so that it is completely covered. Place on a baking tray and bake in a pre-heated oven at 400°F/200°C (Gas Mark 6) for 20 minutes.

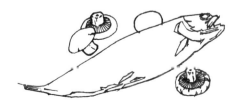

Dolmades

Illustrated opposite page 48.

(Serves 4. Supplies 330 calories and 120mg sodium per portion.)

Imperial (Metric)
8 oz (225g) onion
2 cloves garlic
1 tablespoonful olive oil
1 lb (450g) minced beef (preferably minced steak which has less fat)
1 green pepper, de-seeded and chopped
6 oz (175g) mushrooms, wiped and sliced
1 lb (450g) fresh tomatoes, skinned and chopped
1 bay leaf
1 teaspoonful oregano
Freshly ground black pepper
12 large green cabbage leaves *or* young vine leaves
¼ pint (150ml) water

1. Finely chop the onion and crush the garlic. Cook together in the oil over a low heat for 2 minutes. Add the mince, breaking it up as you do so. Turn up heat and cook, stirring well, until evenly browned.

2. Add the pepper, mushrooms and tomatoes (reserving 2 tablespoonsful chopped tomatoes for stock). Add the herbs and simmer for 45 minutes, stirring occasionally.

3. Set the oven at 325°F/170°C (Gas Mark 3). Have ready a large pan of boiling water and quickly plunge the leaves (in two or three batches if necessary) into the water and blanch for 2 minutes. This makes the leaves easier to roll up.

4. Drain the leaves and divide the filling between them. Place the filling in the centre of the leaf, across the leaf's width. Gently fold the sides over the filling and then fold the top and bottom over. Carefully place each rolled loaf in an oval ovenproof dish, ideally large enough to take all the leaves in one single layer. Pour over the water and add the chopped tomatoes. Cover with foil and bake in the oven for 30 minutes. Serve hot with a little of the cooking stock spooned over.

Scotch Eggs

Illustrated opposite page 49.

(Makes 2. Each supplies 450 calories and 110mg sodium.)

Imperial (Metric)
2 eggs, hard-boiled
3 tablespoonsful wholemeal flour
3 oz (75g) ground hazelnuts
4 oz (100g) low-salt breadcrumbs
Pinch of cayenne pepper
½ teaspoonful thyme
½ teaspoonful sage
Pinch of oregano
2 oz (50g) very finely chopped onion
2 eggs, beaten
2 tablespoonsful oil

1. Heat the oven to 400°F/200°C (Gas Mark 6). Shell the eggs and roll in 1 tablespoonful flour. Set aside.

2. Place the hazelnuts, breadcrumbs, cayenne pepper, thyme, sage, oregano and onion in a bowl. Mix in well till thoroughly blended.

3. Add half the beaten egg to the mixture. Mix in thoroughly. Divide the mix in two and shape each half into a ball.

4. Flatten with the palm of the hand and carefully lay one hard-boiled egg in each ball. Gently work the nut mixture up around the sides of the egg so it is thoroughly covered. Smooth over any cracks.

5. Beat the remaining egg and pour into a shallow bowl. Place the remaining flour in a second bowl. Dip each scotch egg into the beaten egg, making sure it is thoroughly coated. Then gently coat in the flour.

6. Put the oil in a small baking tin and heat in the oven for 2 minutes. Place the eggs in the hot oil and bake in the centre of the oven for 40 minutes, basting occasionally and turning the eggs so they cook evenly. Serve hot or cold.

Pizza

Illustrated opposite page 49.

(Serves 4. Supplies 300 calories and 50mg sodium per portion.)

Tomato Sauce:

Imperial (Metric)
6 oz (175g) onion
2 cloves garlic
1 tablespoonful oil
1 red pepper, de-seeded and chopped
1 lb (450g) fresh tomatoes, skinned
1 teaspoonful oregano or basil
Freshly ground black pepper

Base:

Imperial (Metric)
8 oz (225g) 100 per cent wholemeal flour
½ teaspoonful dried oregano *or* basil
½ oz (13g) low-sodium margarine
¼ pint (150ml) tepid water
½ oz (13g) fresh yeast
25mg vitamin C tablet, crushed

Topping:

Imperial (Metric)
1 green pepper, de-seeded and cut into 1-inch (2.5cm) strips
4 oz (100g) open mushrooms, chopped
4 tablespoonsful sweetcorn kernels (not tinned)

1. Make the tomato sauce. Finely chop the onion, crush the garlic and sauté together in the oil for 2 minutes. Stir in the chopped red pepper and the tomatoes, breaking up the tomatoes with the back of a spoon.

2. Add the herbs and bring to the boil. Reduce heat and continue to cook for 20 minutes. The sauce should be quite thick and pulpy.

3   Place the flour and remaining oregano in a bowl and rub in margarine. Pour tepid water onto the yeast and crushed vitamin C tablet and stir together. Pour onto the flour mixture and, using the hands, draw up to form a dough.

4. Turn out onto a lightly floured surface and knead for 5 minutes until smooth. Cover with an upturned bowl and leave to rest for 10 minutes.

5. Heat the oven to 450°F/230°C (Gas Mark 8). Lightly grease a 10-inch (25cm) flan dish or a baking sheet. When dough is rested roll out to line the flan dish or into a circle 10 inches (25cm) in diameter. Alternatively make four small pizzas. Place in dish or on tray.

6. Smooth tomato sauce over the dough leaving ½-inch (1cm) free around edge. Arrange the pepper, mushroom and sweetcorn on top.

7. Stand in a warm place to let the base rise (about 15 minutes). Bake in the centre of the oven for 15 minutes. If the topping needs a little longer reduce heat to 400°F/200°C (Gas Mark 6) for few minutes more.

Stuffed Marrow Rings

(Serves 4. Supplies 250 calories and 60mg sodium per portion.)

Imperial (Metric)
1 medium-sized marrow or 2 small ones
4 oz (100g) ground nuts
4 oz (100g) low-salt breadcrumbs
4 oz (100g) onion
3 oz (75g) button mushrooms
1 teaspoonful chopped fresh sage *or* ½ teaspoonful dried
½ teaspoonful chopped fresh thyme *or* ¼ teaspoonful dried
Freshly ground black pepper
1 oz (25g) finely grated Cheddar cheese
1 egg, beaten
A little water to bind, if necessary

1. Heat an oven to 350°F/180°C (Gas Mark 4). Cut the marrow into 1-inch (2.5cm) thick rings. Steam for 5 minutes until just tender. Scoop out the seeds using a teaspoon and discard.

2. Prepare the stuffing by mixing all the ingredients together. Add a little water to moisten if needed. Place stuffing in each ring, pressing it in well.

3. Carefully arrange the rings in a shallow ovenproof dish. Pour 3 tablespoonsful of water in the base. Cover with foil and bake for 30 minutes.

Vegetable Pasties

Illustrated opposite page 49.

(Makes 2. Each supplies 350 calories and 12mg sodium.)

Pastry:

Imperial (Metric)
4 oz (100g) 100 per cent wholemeal flour
2 oz (50g) low-sodium margarine
Pinch of thyme
Cold water to mix

Filling:

Imperial (Metric)
10 oz (275g) selected vegetables; choose from carrot, potato, onion,
    swede, turnip, parsnip, button mushrooms, courgette, green pepper
1 tablespoonful salt-free vegetable stock
½ teaspoonful thyme
Freshly ground black pepper
Milk to glaze

1. Rub the margarine into the flour. Stir in the thyme. Chill while preparing
   the filling. Heat the oven to 400°F/200°C (Gas Mark 6).

2. Prepare the vegetables. Dice them evenly and mix with the stock and
   seasonings.

3. Add just enough cold water to mix the pastry to a soft dough. Divide in
   two and roll each out to a rough circle, just over 7 inches (18cm) across.
   Using a 7-inch (18cm) plate as a guide, cut out two circles.

4. Divide the filling between the circles. Arrange it down the middle of the
   circles. Brush the edges with a little cold water. Bring the two sides together
   to meet over the filling and gently press edges together to seal. Flute with
   the back of a knife.

5. Glaze the pasties with a little milk and bake in the centre of the oven for
   20-25 minutes until the filling is soft (gently test with a vegetable knife).
   Serve hot or cold. An ideal packed lunch.

Cod and Mushroom Pie

(Serves 4. Supplies 300 calories and 120mg sodium per portion.)

Imperial (Metric)
1 lb (450g) cod fillet
½ pint (300ml) court bouillon (page 70)
4 oz (100g) button mushrooms
1 dessertspoonful oil
4 oz (100g) onion
2 oz (50g) low-sodium margarine
1 oz (25g) 85 per cent wholemeal flour
¼ pint (150ml) skim milk
1 lb (450g) potatoes
Sprig of mint
2 tablespoonsful skim milk
Knob of unsalted butter
Freshly ground black pepper

1. Wash the cod and put it in a pan with the court bouillon. Poach until cod is just cooked (about 10 minutes). Strain the fish and reserve the stock for making the sauce. When cool enough to handle, skin and remove any bones. Flake fish.

2. Wipe the mushrooms and cut in half. Sauté in the oil for a few minutes. Scrub the potatoes and cut into small pieces. Place in a pan with the mint and just cover with cold water. Bring to the boil, reduce heat and cook for 20 minutes until just soft.

3. Finely chop the onion. Gently cook in the margarine, without browning, for 2 minutes. Stir in the flour. Gradually add the milk and ¼ pint (150ml) of stock reserved from the fish, beating well.

4. Bring the sauce to the boil, then reduce heat. Stir in the mushrooms and fish and season to taste with freshly ground black pepper. Keep warm over a low heat until the potatoes are ready.

5. When the potatoes are cooked, drain and quickly mash with the milk and butter. Season with a little freshly ground black pepper and salt substitute if liked.

6. Heat the grill to red hot. Place the fish mixture in the base of a heatproof dish and top with the mashed potatoes. Spread evenly across top and use a fork to roughen the surface. Grill for 5 minutes or until the top is crunchy and brown.

Macaroni Medley

(Serves 4. Supplies 330 calories and 93mg sodium per portion.)

Imperial (Metric)
1 cauliflower *or* 8 oz (225g) courgettes
5 oz (125g) wholemeal macaroni
4 oz (100g) onion
4 oz (100g) button mushrooms
½ green pepper
1½ oz (38g) low-salt margarine
1½ oz (38g) 85 per cent wholemeal flour
½ pint (300ml) skim milk
4 tablespoonsful fresh or frozen cooked sweetcorn kernels
Pinch of dried thyme
Freshly ground black pepper
1 oz (25g) grated Cheddar cheese
1 tablespoonful sesame seeds

1. Divide the cauliflower into florets or cut the courgettes into ½-inch (1cm) slices. Steam or lightly boil until just tender. Reserve ¼ pint (150ml) of the cooking liquid.

2. Plunge the pasta into boiling water. Cook until just soft and set aside.

3. Finely chop the onion. Wipe and halve the mushrooms and de-seed the pepper.

4. Melt the margarine in a large pan and gently cook the chopped onion, without browning, over a low heat until soft (about 8 minutes).

5. Stir in the flour and mix to a smooth paste. Cook for 1 minute, then gradually add the milk and stock. Bring to the boil so the sauce can thicken.

6. Add the mushrooms, pepper and sweetcorn and simmer for 5 minutes. Add the thyme and some freshly ground black pepper to taste.

7. Pre-heat a grill to red hot. Add the pasta and cauliflower or courgettes and stir in together. Pile into a heatproof dish. Sprinkle over the cheese and sesame seeds and grill for a few minutes until golden-brown.

Coley and Courgette Braise

(Serves 4. Supplies 200 calories and 130mg sodium per portion.)

Imperial (Metric)
1 lb (450g) coley
12 oz (325g) courgettes
6 oz (175g) button mushrooms
1 large onion
2 cloves garlic
1 tablespoonful sunflower oil
15 oz (425g) tin tomatoes *or* 1 lb (450g) fresh
1 teaspoonful oregano
½ pint (300ml) dry cider
1 tablespoonful cornflour
Freshly ground black pepper

1. Light the oven and heat to 400°F/200°C (Gas Mark 6). Wash and skin the coley and cut into 2-inch (5cm) cubes.

2. Wash the courgettes and slice. Wipe mushrooms and slice. Place coley, courgettes and mushrooms in ovenproof dish.

3. Finely chop the onion and crush the garlic. Sauté both together in the oil for two minutes without browning.

4. Stir the tomatoes into the pan and add the oregano and cider. Bring to the boil then pour over fish and vegetables. Cover with foil and bake for 30 minutes. Blend cornflour with a little cold water and add to dish to thicken sauce. Return to oven for further 5 minutes. Season with black pepper and serve.

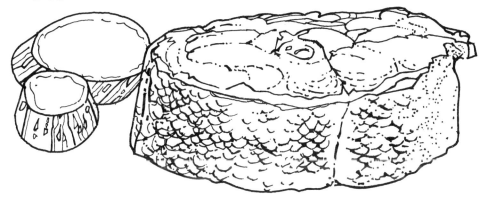

Chilli Beans

(Serves 4. Supplies 275 calories and 130mg sodium per portion.)

Imperial (Metric)
8 oz (225g) onion
8 oz (225g) carrots
3 green chillies
2 tablespoonsful oil
2 × 15 oz (425g) tins tomatoes *or* 2 lb (900g) fresh
¼ pint (150ml) water
8 oz (225g) red kidney beans, soaked overnight
1 green pepper, de-seeded and chopped
1 red pepper, de-seeded and chopped
½ teaspoonful ground cumin
Freshly ground black pepper

1. Finely chop the onion and carrot. De-seed and very finely chop the green chillies.

2. Cook the onion, carrot and chillies in the oil over a low heat for 2 minutes.

3. Stir in the tomatoes, water, beans and chopped peppers and cumin and bring to the boil.

4. Cover, reduce the heat and simmer over a very low heat for 2½-3 hours until the beans are just soft. Add more water if necessary. Alternatively transfer mixture to a pre-heated oven, 375°F/190°C (Gas Mark 5) to cook.

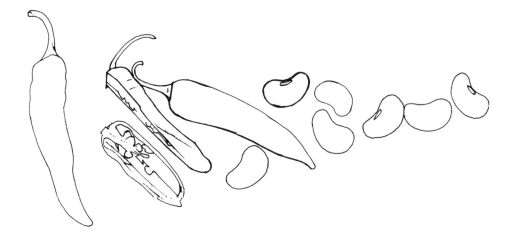

Chicken Dopiaza

(Serves 4. Supplies 190 calories and 100mg sodium per portion.)

Imperial (Metric)
2 large onions
2 green chillies
1 tablespoonful sunflower oil
1 tablespoonful root ginger, grated
3 teaspoonsful ground coriander
2 teaspoonsful ground cumin
1 teaspoonful cumin seeds
2 teaspoonsful turmeric
1 teaspoonful ground cardamom
4 chicken breasts, skinned
½ lb (225g) fresh tomatoes, skinned
4 tablespoonsful water
1 tablespoonful unsalted tomato purée
1 green pepper, de-seeded and chopped
2 tablespoonsful yogurt

1. Finely chop the onions and de-seed and finely chop the chillies. Cook in the oil over a low heat for 2 minutes. Stir in the spices. Continue to cook for a further 2 minutes.

2. Add the chicken to the pan. Cook for a few seconds first on one side and then turn over to cook evenly.

3. Add the tomatoes, water, tomato purée and the pepper. Bring to the boil, then reduce heat. Cover pan tightly and cook for 50 minutes.

4. Turn the chicken during cooking. Just before serving stir in the yogurt. Pour the sauce over the chicken on a serving plate.

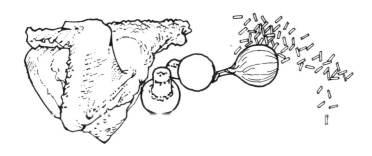

Mushroom Quiche

(Serves 4. Supplies 380 calories and 80mg sodium per portion.)

Pastry:

Imperial (Metric)
6 oz (175g) wholemeal flour
3 oz (75g) low sodium margarine
Cold water to mix

Filling:

Imperial (Metric)
2 cloves garlic
4 oz (100g) onion
1 tablespoonful oil
6 oz (175g) button mushrooms
1 teaspoonful fresh thyme, chopped, *or* ½ teaspoonful dried
Freshly ground black pepper
2 free-range eggs
⅓ pint (200ml) natural yogurt

1. Sieve the flour into a bowl and rub in the margarine until the mixture resembles fine breadcrumbs. Add sufficient cold water to mix to a dough. Roll out and line an 8-inch (20cm) flan dish. Bake blind at 400°F/200°C (Gas Mark 6) for 10 minutes.

2. Meanwhile prepare the filling. Crush the garlic and finely chop the onion. Cook gently in the oil for 4 minutes without browning.

3. Wipe and finely chop the mushrooms. Add to the pan and stir in well. Cook 2 minutes.

4. Beat the herbs with eggs, and yogurt and season with pepper.

5. When the flan case is ready, spread the onion and mushroom mixture evenly in the base. Pour over the egg mixture. Bake in the centre of the oven for 25-30 minutes until golden-brown and set. Serve hot or cold.

Khichhari

(Serves 4. Supplies 370 calories and 72mg sodium per portion.)

Imperial (Metric)
8 oz (225g) carrots
8 oz (225g) onions
2 cloves garlic
1 tablespoonful oil
1 teaspoonful cumin seeds
1½ teaspoonsful ground coriander
1 teaspoonful garam masala
1 teaspoonful turmeric
Pinch of paprika
Pinch of nutmeg
8 oz (225g) long-grain brown rice
1¾ pints (1 litre) water
6 oz (175g) red lentils
Freshly ground black pepper

1. Finely dice the carrots and onions. Crush the garlic. Sauté together in the oil over a low heat for 2 minutes.

2. Stir in the spices and mix in well. Cook for 1 minute before stirring in the rice. Cook for a further 2 minutes to coat the grains of rice. Pour on the water and the lentils. Bring to the boil, reduce heat and cover.

3. Cook for 30-35 minutes until the rice and lentils are just soft. Check during cooking to make sure the mixture doesn't become too dry.

4. If, at the end of cooking, some fluid still remains turn up the heat and cook quickly until all the moisture has evaporated. Season with pepper and serve.

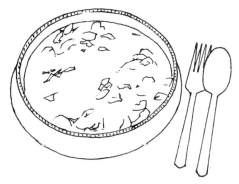

Leek Soufflé Quiche

(Serves 4. Supplies 270 calories and 60mg sodium per portion.)

Pastry:

Imperial (Metric)
4 oz (100g) 100 per cent wholemeal flour
2 oz (50g) low-sodium margarine
Cold water to mix

Filling:

Imperial (Metric)
8 oz (225g) leeks
½ oz (13g) low-sodium margarine
½ oz (13g) 85 per cent wholewheat flour
¼ pint (150ml) skim milk
2 eggs, separated
Pinch of rosemary
Freshly ground black pepper

1. Heat the oven to 400°F/200°C (Gas Mark 6). Rub the margarine into the flour until mixture resembles fine breadcrumbs. Add sufficient cold water to mix to a dough. Roll out and line a 7-inch (18cm) flan ring.

2. Line with greaseproof and baking beans and bake in the centre of the oven for 10 minutes. Remove the beans and paper and continue to bake for a further 5 minutes.

3. While flan is baking, prepare the filling. Trim the leeks and cut into ¼-inch (5mm) thick slices. Plunge into boiling water and cook quickly for 5 minutes. Drain.

4. Melt the margarine in a pan and stir in the flour. Gradually add the milk, beating well to make a smooth sauce, bring to the boil and then quickly pour onto the egg yolks. Beat well. Stir in the leeks. Season with rosemary and pepper.

5. When the flan case is ready, stiffly whisk the egg whites. Gently fold them into the leek sauce with a metal spoon. Pour into the flan case and gently smooth over the top. Bake in the centre of the oven for 20-25 minutes until well-risen but just firm to the touch. Serve hot.

Opposite: Dolmades (page 36) make a stunning dinner party dish.

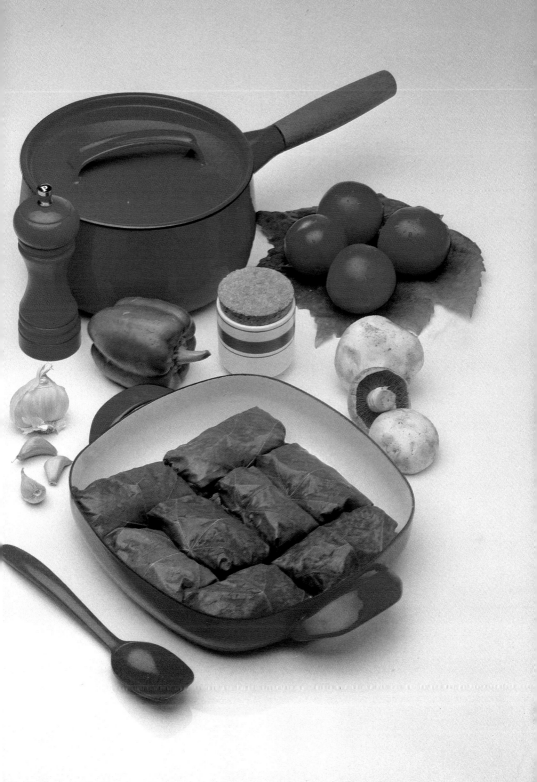

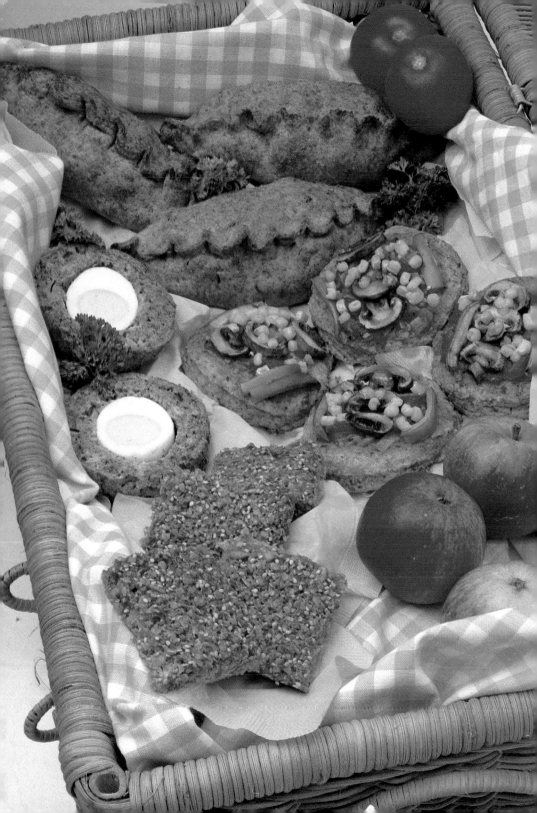

Almond and Mushroom Bake

(Serves 4. Supplies 390 calories and 45mg sodium per portion.)

Imperial (Metric)
6 oz (175g) almonds
6 oz (175g) breadcrumbs
6 oz (175g) button mushrooms
½ teaspoonful lemon rind, finely grated
1 tablespoonful chopped parsley
½ teaspoonful thyme
1 small onion, finely chopped
Freshly ground black pepper
2 eggs
A little salt-free stock to moisten

1. Put the almonds into a liquidizer and grind finely. Mix together with the breadcrumbs. Lightly grease a small loaf tin. Heat the oven to 375°F/190°C (Gas Mark 5).

2. Wipe and finely chop the mushrooms. Add to the nut and breadcrumbs with the seasonings and finely chopped onion.

3. Beat the eggs together and add to bowl. Using a fork, mix in the eggs adding a little stock if required. The mixture should be moist but not soggy.

4. Press the mixture into the prepared tin. Smooth over top and cover with foil. Bake in the centre of the oven for 45 minutes. Serve sliced, hot or cold.

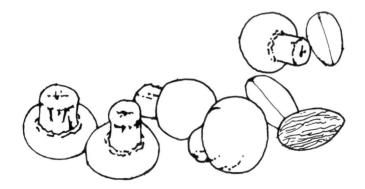

Opposite: Pack up a picnic with Vegetable Pasties (page 40); Scotch Eggs (page 37); individual Pizzas (page 38); Sesame Flapjacks (page 83).

Lamb's Liver Casserole

(Serves 4. Supplies 290 calories and 190mg sodium per portion.)

Imperial (Metric)
8 oz (225g) onions
8 oz (225g) carrots
½ green pepper
8 oz (225g) swede
2 sticks celery
1 lb (450g) lamb's liver
2 tablespoonsful wholemeal flour
Freshly ground black pepper
1 small eating apple
Pinch of thyme
2 teaspoonsful fresh sage, finely chopped
1½ pints (900ml) water
1 tablespoonful cornflour

1. Finely slice the onions and carrots and chop the green pepper. Peel and dice the swede and finely chop the celery. Place the prepared vegetables in the base of a casserole dish.

2. Wash the liver and cut into 2-inch (5cm) strips. Mix the flour with a little freshly ground black pepper and place in a shallow dish. Toss the liver strips in the flour mixture and then place in the casserole.

3. Peel, core and dice the apple and add to the casserole. Sprinkle herbs over and pour on the water. Place in a pre-heated oven at 400°F/200°C (Gas Mark 6) for 2 hours. 5 minutes before the end of cooking time blend the cornflour with a little cold water and add to the casserole to thicken the gravy. Return to the oven for a final few minutes cooking.

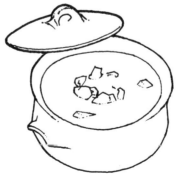

Haricot Goulash

(Serves 4. Supplies 240 calories and 106mg sodium per portion.)

Imperial (Metric)
2 cloves garlic
8 oz (225g) onion
2 sticks celery
8 oz (225g) carrots
1 tablespoonful oil
1 tablespoonful paprika
2 × 15 oz (425g) tins tomatoes
1 pint (600ml) water
8 oz (225g) haricot beans, soaked overnight
1 green pepper, de-seeded and chopped
1 red pepper, de-seeded and chopped
½ teaspoonful oregano
2 bay leaves
Freshly ground black pepper

1. Crush the garlic; finely chop the onion, celery and carrots and sauté together with the garlic in the oil for 2 minutes without browning.

2. Stir in the paprika and cook for a further minute.

3. Add the tomatoes, water, beans and chopped peppers and herbs. Bring to the boil and either cover the pan, reduce the heat and continue cooking on top of the hob for 2-2¼ hours or transfer to a casserole dish and cook in a preheated oven 375°F/190°C (Gas Mark 5). Add more water if necessary during cooking. Season to taste with black pepper and serve with brown rice and a green salad.

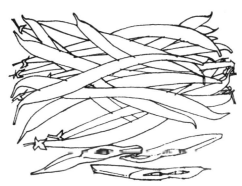

Curried Cauliflower and Cashew Rice

(Serves 2. Supplies 450 calories and 100mg sodium per portion.)

Imperial (Metric)
1 large onion
1 stick celery
1 clove of garlic
4 oz (100g) carrots
1 tablespoonful oil
1 teaspoonful turmeric
1 teaspoonful ground coriander
1 teaspoonful ground cumin
½ teaspoonful cumin seeds
4 oz (100g) long-grain brown rice
¾ pint (450ml) water or salt-free vegetable stock
4 oz (100g) mushrooms, sliced
1 cauliflower, broken into florets
1 green or red pepper
2 oz (50g) cashew nuts
Freshly ground black pepper

1. Finely chop the onion and celery, crush the garlic and scrub and finely dice the carrot. Sauté all together in the oil over a low heat for a few minutes, without browning.

2. Add the turmeric, coriander, ground cumin and cumin seeds to the pan and stir in thoroughly. Cook for 2 minutes. Stir in the rice and cook gently until evenly coated in the mixture.

3. Add the water or stock, mushrooms and cauliflower florets and bring to the boil. Reduce heat and cover. Cook for 30-40 minutes until the rice is just soft and all the liquid has been absorbed. Just before serving stir in the cashew nuts and season with freshly ground black pepper.

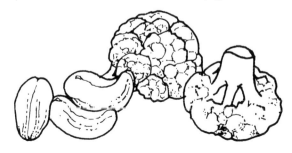

Walnut Patties

(Makes 4. Each supplies 280 calories and 30mg sodium.)

Imperial (Metric)
2 oz (50g) walnut pieces
1 oz (25g) ground hazelnuts
3 oz (75g) low-sodium breadcrumbs
2 oz (50g) onion
1 small stick celery
1 tablespoonful oil
3 oz (75g) finely grated carrots
1 teaspoonful dried thyme *or* 2 teaspoonsful fresh
2 tablespoonsful 'no-added-salt' tomato purée
1 free-range egg, beaten
Freshly ground black pepper
Oil for cooking

1. Grind the walnuts in a blender. Mix with the hazelnuts and breadcrumbs (reserving 2 tablespoonsful of breadcrumbs).

2. Finely chop the onion and celery and sauté both in the oil for 3 minutes.

3. Add the onion mixture to the breadcrumb mixture with the carrots, thyme, tomato purée and egg. Mix together well. Divide into 4 equal portions and shape each into a burger shape. Coat in the extra breadcrumbs and chill for at least 30 minutes.

4. Heat a little oil in a large frying pan. Cook the patties for a few minutes on each side. Drain off surplus oil and serve.

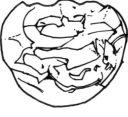
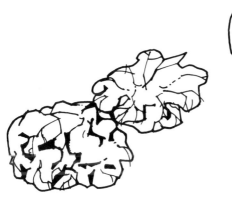

Summer Pie

(Serves 4. Supplies 450 calories and 40mg sodium per portion.)

Flaky Pastry:

Imperial (Metric)
8 oz (225g) wholemeal flour
6 oz (175g) unsalted butter
2 teaspoonsful lemon juice
6-8 tablespoonsful cold water

Filling:

Imperial (Metric)
4 oz (100g) onion
2 cloves garlic
1 lb (450g) fresh tomatoes
1 lb (450g) courgettes
Freshly ground black pepper
2 teaspoonsful fresh basil *or* 1 teaspoonful dried
Cornflour to thicken
Beaten egg to glaze

1. Sieve flour into bowl and add bran from the sieve to the bowl. Divide the butter into four and rub one quarter into the flour, until the mixture resembles fine breadcrumbs. Return the remaining fat to the fridge.

2. Add the lemon juice and 6 tablespoonsful water. With a knife mix to a soft dough, adding extra 2 tablespoonsful water if required. The dough should be soft. Knead lightly to make it smooth and silky but do not be heavy-handed.

3. Form the dough into a rough rectangle and place on a lightly-floured surface. Carefully roll it out to an oblong about 5 × 15 inches (12 × 38cm). Take the second quarter of fat from the fridge and place it, in little dabs, on the top two-thirds of the dough. Fold the lower, empty third up over the centre third and fold the top third down. Seal the edges and place in the refrigerator, covered, to rest for 20 minutes.

4. Take the dough out of the fridge and place on the surface so that the smaller edges of the rectangle are parallel with you. Roll out and fold as before. Repeat for the last of the fat and then roll and fold one final time without the addition of fat. Remember to rest the dough inbetween.

5. While the dough is resting in the fridge after the third rolling and folding, start to prepare the filling. Finely chop the onion and crush the garlic. Sauté together gently in the oil, without browning.

6. While the onion and garlic are cooking, peel the tomatoes by plunging them into a bowl of boiling water. Remove after 1 minute; the skins should come away easily. Roughly chop and add to the pan.

7. Slice the courgettes and add to the pan with the basil. Bring to the boil, cover and reduce heat. Simmer for 20 minutes.

8. At end of cooking time, season to taste and if mixture is quite thin thicken with a little cornflour blended with cold water.

9. Place the courgette mixture in the base of an 8-inch (20cm) pie dish. Roll out the pastry into a circle 9 inches (23cm) in diameter. The pastry will be about ¼-inch (5mm) thick. Cut a strip ½-inch (1cm) from around the edge and place on the rim of the dish tucking to make it fit.

10. Brush with water and then carefully lift the remaining pastry onto the dish. Trim the edges and press lightly together to seal. Knock the edges up with the back of a knife; this helps the edges to flake up.

11. Roll out strips from the pastry trimmings and cut into leaf shapes. Arrange on top of pie. Glaze with beaten egg and bake for 35 minutes in a pre-heated oven at 425°F/220°C (Gas Mark 7).

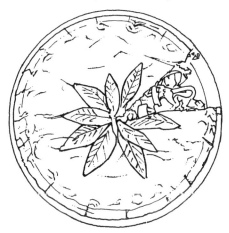

Pancakes Stuffed with Spinach

(Serves 4. Supplies 280 calories and 180mg sodium per portion.)

Batter:

Imperial (Metric)
4 oz (100g) wholemeal flour
1 egg
¼ pint (150ml) milk and water, mixed
Vegetable oil

Filling:

Imperial (Metric)
1 lb (450g) fresh or frozen spinach

Sauce:

Imperial (Metric)
1 onion
1½ oz (38g) low-salt margarine
1 oz (25g) wholemeal flour
¼ pint (150ml) skim milk
¼ pint (150ml) cold water
6 oz (175g) mushrooms
½ teaspoonful lemon juice
Freshly ground black pepper

1. Sieve the flour into a bowl and add back the bran from the sieve. Make a well in the centre and add the egg. Beat in and then gradually add half the milk and water mixture. Beat thoroughly for several minutes (this is easiest with a hand whisk). Add the remaining fluid for the batter and set aside.

2. Wash the spinach thoroughly if using fresh. Remove any coarse stalks and put it in a pan with just the water that clings to the leaves. Cook for few minutes until tender. Finely chop and squeeze out as much moisture as possible.

3. Heat a little oil in a 7-inch (18cm) pancake pan. Tip in just enough mixture
    to coat the base of the pan and cook gently until set. Toss or turn to cook
    the other side. When ready, keep the pancakes warm on a plate and cook
    the rest of the batter in the same way, keeping each pancake hot.

4. Finely chop the onion and sauté in the margarine until soft. Stir in the flour
    and then gradually add the milk and water. Bring to the boil, then reduce
    heat and add the mushrooms with the lemon juice and a little seasoning.
    Heat through on a low heat while preparing the pancakes.

5. Place a little cooked spinach along the centre of each pancake. Roll up
    tightly and transfer them to an ovenproof dish. Arrange the pancakes in
    the dish and, when all have been filled, pour over the mushroom sauce.
    Cover with foil and bake in a pre-heated oven at 375°F/190°C (Gas Mark
    5) for 20 minutes to heat through.

Lamb Kebabs

(Serves 4. Supplies 500 calories and 70mg sodium per portion.)

Imperial (Metric)
1 lb (450g) lamb fillet
Juice of 1 lemon
3 tablespoonsful olive oil
Freshly ground black pepper
2 courgettes
2 large tomatoes
1 green pepper

1. Put the lamb in a shallow dish. Mix together the lemon juice, olive oil and
    freshly ground black pepper and pour it over the lamb. Cover with cling
    film, put in the fridge and leave to marinate for at least 3 hours. Turn the
    meat several times.

2. Cut the lamb into 1-inch (2.5cm) chunks. Cut the courgettes into ½-inch
    (1cm) slices, quarter the tomatoes and de-seed the pepper and cut into
    thick strips.

3. Thread alternative chunks of meat, courgettes, tomato and pepper onto
    skewers. Place on a wire rack and baste with any surplus marinade. Either
    barbecue or cook under a red hot grill for 20-25 minutes until the meat
    is just cooked. Serve with salads.

Summer Chicken Risotto

(Serves 4. Supplies 320 calories and 100mg sodium per portion.)

Imperial (Metric)
4 chicken joints (boned breast is best)
4 oz (100g) onion
2 cloves garlic
4 oz (100g) carrots
1 tablespoonful olive oil
8 oz (225g) long-grain brown rice
1½ pints (900ml) vegetable stock
1 teaspoonful fresh thyme *or* ½ teaspoonful dried
4 tablespoonsful sweetcorn kernels
8 oz (225g) courgettes
1 green pepper
3 oz (75g) cashew nuts
Freshly ground black pepper

1. Skin the joints and cut the flesh away from the bones. Cut into bite-sized pieces.

2. Finely chop the onion, crush the garlic and finely dice the carrots. Sauté in the oil for a few minutes without browning. Stir in the rice and cook for 1 minute so the grains become transparent. Add the stock, thyme, sweetcorn and chicken pieces. Bring to the boil, cover and reduce heat. Cook for 10 minutes.

3. While cooking, chop the courgettes. After 10 minutes add to the pan. Cover and continue cooking until rice is just soft. Meanwhile chop the pepper. At end of cooking add pepper and cashew nuts to the pan. Stir in well and turn up heat to evaporate any excess moisture. Season with black pepper and serve.

6.

VEGETABLES AND SALADS

Mixed Bean Salad

Illustrated opposite page 64.

(Serves 4. Supplies 145 calories and 12mg sodium per portion.)

Imperial (Metric)
4 oz (100g) black-eye beans*
8 oz (225g) French beans
2 tablespoonsful sunflower oil
1 tablespoonful fresh lemon juice
2 spring onions
Freshly ground black pepper

1. Place the black-eye beans in a pan of cold water. Bring to the boil, reduce the heat and simmer for 45-50 minutes until just soft.

2. While the beans are cooking, top and tail the French beans and cut into 2-inch (5cm) long pieces. Plunge into a little boiling water, or steam, for 8-10 minutes until just soft. Time the cooking so that both beans finish cooking together.

3. While the beans are cooking, prepare the dressing. Place the oil and lemon juice in a screw top jar. Trim the spring onions and chop finely. Add to the jar with the pepper.

4. Strain the beans thoroughly and place in a bowl. Vigorously shake the dressing ingredients together so they are well blended and pour over the beans. Leave to cool before serving.

* Black-eye beans, unlike other dried beans do not need soaking before cooking.

Tossed Green Salad

(Enough for 5 or 6. Supplies around 50 calories and 5mg sodium per portion.)

Imperial (Metric)
1 Cos or Webb's Wonder lettuce *or* 2 small round lettuce
½ a cucumber
1 green pepper
2 spring onions
2 tablespoonsful olive oil
1 teaspoonful white wine vinegar
Freshly ground black pepper
Pinch of mustard powder

1. Remove any discoloured outer leaves from the lettuce. Carefully wash the good leaves and shake to remove excess moisture.

2. Finely slice the cucumber. De-seed and slice the pepper into rings. Arrange the lettuce, cucumber and pepper in a large salad bowl.

3. Finely chop the spring onions. Place in a screw top jar with the oil and vinegar, pepper and mustard powder. Shake together vigorously and pour over the lettuce. Serve at once.

Swede Purée

(Serves 5. Supplies 65 calories and 110mg sodium per portion.)

Imperial (Metric)
1½ lb (675g) swede
8 oz (225g) carrots
1 bay leaf
½ oz (13g) low-salt margarine or unsalted butter
2 tablespoonsful skim milk
Freshly ground black pepper

1. Peel the swede and cut into chunks. Scrub and dice the carrots. Place in a large pan with cold water and the bay leaf. Bring to the boil, then cover, reduce heat and simmer for 40 minutes.

2. Drain and add the margarine and milk. Mash together thoroughly or rub through a sieve for a very smooth result. Season to taste with black pepper.

Spicy Potato with Carrot

(Serves 4. Supplies 135 calories and 50mg sodium per portion.)

Imperial (Metric)
8 oz (225g) potatoes
6 oz (175g) carrots
6 oz (175g) onion
2 tablespoonsful oil
1 ½ teaspoonsful cumin seeds
Freshly ground black pepper
1 spring onion, finely chopped

1. Scrub the potatoes. Cook for 15-20 minutes until tender. Drain and chop.

2. Scrub the carrots and dice finely. Finely chop the onion.

3. Heat the oil in large frying pan. Add the cumin seeds and let them sizzle for 1 minute. Stir in the carrot and onion. Cook over a low heat for 10 minutes, without browning, turning so they cook evenly.

4. Stir in the chopped potatoes and heat through. Season with pepper and stir in the chopped spring onion. Serve at once.

Cabbage Sauté

(Serves 4. Supplies 90 calories and 10mg sodium per portion.)

Imperial (Metric)
1 lb (450g) white cabbage
1 onion, chopped
1 tablespoonful oil
½ oz (13g) unsalted butter
Freshly ground black pepper
½ teaspoonful caraway seeds (optional)

1. Wash the cabbage and shred finely. Plunge into boiling water and cook for 3 minutes. Meanwhile sauté the chopped onion in the oil and butter over a low heat, without browning.

2. Drain the cabbage and add to the onion. Stir together well and continue to cook for a further 2 minutes. Stir in the seeds if using and season liberally with freshly ground black pepper. Serve at once.

Ratatouille

(Serves 5. Supplies 105 calories and 11mg sodium per portion.)

Imperial (Metric)
1 lb (450g) aubergines
8 oz (225g) onions
4 cloves garlic
2 tablespoonsful olive oil
Basil *or* marjoram, 1 dessertspoonful fresh *or* 1 teaspoonful dried
1 lb (450g) courgettes
1 lb (450g) tomatoes
1 green pepper
Freshly ground black pepper

1. Dice the aubergines. Finely chop the onions and crush the garlic. Cook together in the oil over a low heat for 10 minutes, without browning.

2. Meanwhile, wipe and slice the courgettes and skin and chop the tomatoes. De-seed and chop the pepper.

3. Add the prepared vegetables to the pan with the herbs and cover and cook for 45 minutes, stirring occasionally. Season with freshly ground black pepper and serve hot or cold.

Aubergine Curried with Spinach and Potato

(Serves 4. Supplies 140 calories and 70mg sodium per portion.)

Imperial (Metric)
8 oz (225g) aubergine
8 oz (225g) potato
2 tomatoes
4 oz (100g) onion
2 green chillies
8 oz (225g) spinach
2 tablespoonsful sunflower oil
1 teaspoonful grated ginger
1 teaspoonful ground cumin
½ teaspoonful turmeric
1 tablespoonful cold water
Freshly ground black pepper

1. Dice the aubergine and potato. Skin the tomatoes and chop the flesh. Finely chop the onion. De-seed and finely chop the chillies. Wash the spinach and chop roughly.

2. Put the oil into a large pan. Add the diced potato and fry until golden.

3. Remove the potato from the pan and add the aubergine. Cook for 2 minutes, then add the onion, ginger, cumin and turmeric. Cook for 1 minute then stir in the tomatoes, water and spinach. Return the potato to the pan.

4. Cook for 15-20 minutes over a low heat, covered, until spinach is soft. Add a little more water if the mixture looks like sticking. Turn up the heat at end of cooking to evaporate any excess moisture.

Spicy French Beans

(Serves 4. Supplies 85 calories and 6mg sodium per portion.)

Imperial (Metric)
1 lb (450g) French beans
4 cloves garlic
½-inch (1cm) cube fresh ginger, grated
6 fl oz (180ml) cold water
2 tablespoonsful olive oil
1½ teaspoonsful cumin seeds
½ teaspoonful chilli powder
1½ teaspoonsful ground coriander
2 tomatoes, skinned and chopped
1 teaspoonful lemon juice
1 teaspoonful ground cumin
Freshly ground black pepper

1. Top and tail the beans and cut into 2-inch (5cm) lengths.

2. Crush the garlic and mince with the ginger, or put both, with half the water, in a liquidizer and blend until smooth.

3. Put the oil into a large pan and add the cumin seeds, chilli powder and ginger and garlic mixture. Stir together and heat for 1 minute.

4. Add the coriander, tomatoes and beans and the remaining water. Stir together well. Cover and simmer for 10 minutes.

5. Add the lemon juice, cumin and some freshly ground black pepper and continue cooking until the mixture is thick.

Chilled Rice Ring

(Serves 6 as a salad accompaniment. Supplies 130 calories and 9mg sodium per portion.)

Imperial (Metric)
6 oz (175g) long-grain brown rice
2 spring onions
1 red pepper
1 green pepper
2 oz (50g) button mushrooms
1 oz (25g) sultanas
2-inch (5cm) piece cucumber
Smear of vegetable oil
Pinch of thyme

1. Put the rice in a pan of cold water and bring to the boil. Reduce heat and cover. Simmer for 25-35 minutes until rice is just tender. Drain.

2. While the rice is cooking, prepare the vegetables. Trim and finely chop the onions. Core and de-seed the peppers and chop. Wipe the mushrooms and chop finely. Sort through the sultanas and discard any stalks. Dice the cucumber.

3. When the rice is cooked and drained mix in the prepared vegetables immediately.

4. Smear oil around an 8-inch (20cm) ring mould and pack the rice mixture in tightly. Cover with cling film and chill for at least 1 hour.

5. When ready to serve invert plate on top of mould and turn out. Fill the centre with some sliced tomatoes or other salad ingredients.

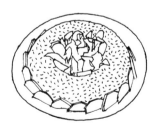

Opposite: Sophisticated salads. From the top: Courgette and Cauliflower Pasta Salad (page 67); Mixed Bean Salad (page 59); Cucumber and Grape Salad (page 66).

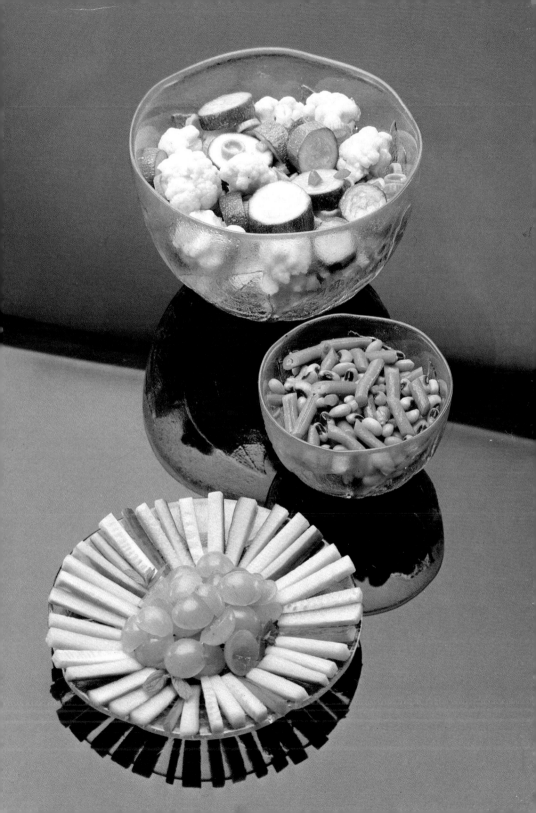

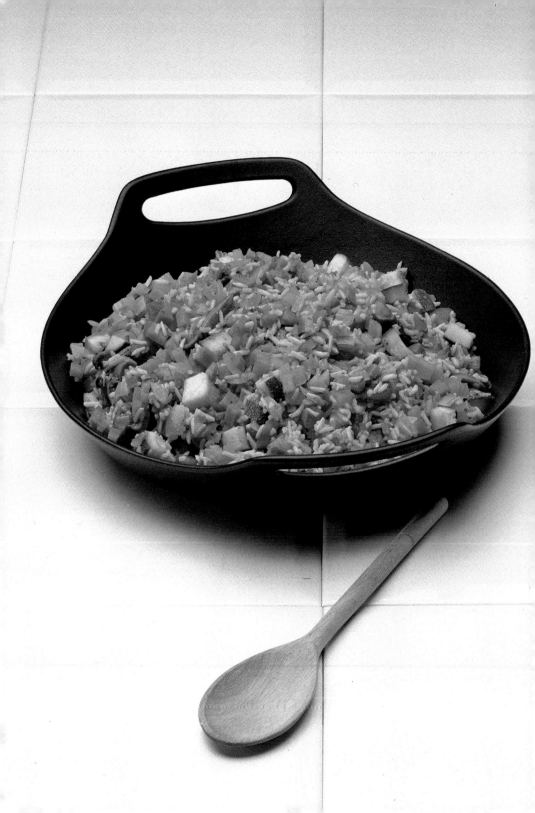

Tangy Mushroom Salad

(Serves 4. Supplies 75 calories and 5mg sodium per portion.)

Imperial (Metric)
6 oz (175g) button mushrooms
2 tablespoonsful olive oil
1 tablespoonful fresh lemon juice
1 tablespoonful chopped chives
1 teaspoonful fresh thyme
Freshly ground black pepper

1. Wipe the mushrooms and slice finely. Arrange in a shallow bowl.

2. In a screwtop jar, put the oil, lemon juice, chives, thyme and black pepper and shake vigorously together. Pour over the mushrooms and toss thoroughly. Chill before serving.

Potato Salad

(Serves 3. Supplies 180 calories and 55mg sodium per portion.)

Imperial (Metric)
12 oz (325g) new potatoes
Sprig of mint
2 tablespoonsful olive oil
1 dessertspoonful white wine vinegar
Pinch of dried thyme
Freshly ground black pepper
4 spring onions
2 tablespoonsful natural yogurt

1. Wash the potatoes to remove any dirt. Place in a pan of cold water with the mint and bring to the boil. Reduce heat and simmer until just soft.

2. While the potatoes are cooking, put the oil, vinegar, thyme and a little black pepper in a screwtop jar and shake vigorously.

3. When the potatoes are ready, drain them and immediately pour over dressing. Leave to get cold.

4. When the potatoes are cold, chop the onions finely and mix with the potatoes. Pour over the yogurt and toss together thoroughly.

Opposite: Rich Vegetable Sauce (page 72) makes a delicious risotto when mixed with brown rice and courgettes.

Coleslaw

(Serves 5. Supplies 115 calories and 40mg sodium per portion.)

Imperial (Metric)
12 oz (325g) white cabbage
6 oz (175g) carrots
4 spring onions
1½ tablespoonsful mayonnaise (page 75)

1. Wash the cabbage and remove the stalky core. Finely shred or grate the cabbage. Scrub the carrots and then grate.

2. Mix the carrots with the cabbage. Finely chop the spring onions and stir in. Mix in the mayonnaise and, if liked, season with a little freshly ground black pepper.

Cucumber and Grape Salad

Illustrated opposite page 64.

(Serves 3. Supplies 70 calories and 5mg sodium per portion.)

Imperial (Metric)
2-inch (5cm) piece of cucumber
4 oz (100g) seedless white grapes
1 tablespoonful olive oil
1 teaspoonful white wine vinegar
1 mint leaf, very finely chopped
Pinch of mustard powder
Freshly ground black pepper

1. Cut the cucumber in two and then cut into fine julienne strips.

2. Wash the grapes and mix with the cucumber sticks.

3. In a screwtop jar, place the oil, vinegar, mint, mustard and a little black pepper. Shake together vigorously and pour over the cucumber and grapes. Chill well before serving.

Courgette and Cauliflower Pasta Salad

Illustrated opposite page 64.

(Serves 4. Supplies 180 calories and 6mg sodium per portion.)

Imperial (Metric)
4 oz (100g) wholemeal pasta spirals or hoops
8 oz (225g) cauliflower florets
8 oz (225g) courgettes, sliced
2 spring onions
2 tablespoonsful oil
1 teaspoonful cider vinegar
Freshly ground black pepper
Pinch of dried thyme
1 green pepper, finely chopped

1. Cook the pasta in boiling water for 12 minutes. After 7 minutes, plunge the cauliflower and courgettes into a separate pan of boiling water (or steam) for 4 minutes.

2. While the vegetables are cooking, put the finely chopped spring onions, and the oil and vinegar with the pepper and thyme in a screwtop jar. Shake vigorously together.

3. When the vegetables and pasta are cooked, drain them and toss immediately in the dressing. Add the chopped pepper. Leave to cool before serving.

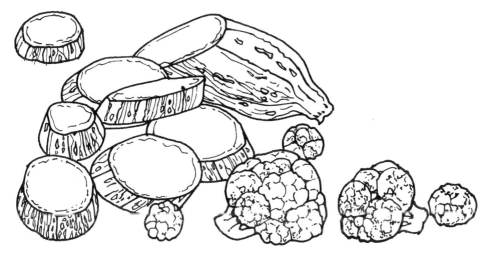

Mushroom and Okra Rice

(Serves 4. Supplies 225 calories and 60mg sodium per portion.)

Imperial (Metric)
6 oz (175g) mushrooms
4 oz (100g) okra
1 large onion
1 tablespoonful oil
1 teaspoonful turmeric
8 oz (225g) long-grain brown rice
1½ pints (900ml) water
1 red pepper, de-seeded and chopped
Freshly ground black pepper

1. Wipe and slice the mushrooms. Wipe the okra and trim each end. Cut into ½-inch (1cm) lengths. Finely chop the onion.

2. Cook the chopped onion in the oil over a low heat for 2 minutes. Stir in the rice and cook gently until all the grains are coated.

3. Add the water and bring to the boil. Stir in prepared mushrooms and okra. Cover and reduce heat and cook for 20 minutes.

4. Add the chopped red pepper and continue to cook for a further 5-10 minutes, depending on the consistency of the rice. The rice should be just soft. If any liquid remains in the pan turn up heat and cook quickly to drive off moisture. Season with pepper and serve.

7.

STOCKS, SAUCES AND DRESSINGS

Vegetable Stock

Imperial (Metric)
1 stick celery
1 onion
2 oz (50g) carrots
6 black peppercorns
1 sprig of fresh thyme
2 bay leaves
3 parsley stalks
2 pints (1.2 litres) water

1. Scrub the celery and roughly chop. Chop the onion and carrots.

2. Place the vegetables with the peppercorns, thyme, bay leaves and parsley with the water in a large saucepan.

3. Cover, bring to the boil then reduce heat and simmer for 1 hour. Alternatively pressure cook for 15 minutes at 15 lb (6 kilos) pressure. Strain off the vegetables. The stock is now ready to use.

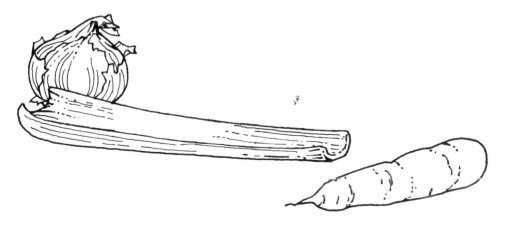

Chicken Stock

Imperial (Metric)
1 chicken carcass
2 pints (1.2 litres) water
1 onion
4 oz (100g) carrots
1 stick celery
2 bay leaves
1 sprig of fresh thyme *or* ½ teaspoonful dried
6 black peppercorns

1. Place the chicken carcass in a large saucepan with the water.

2. Peel and quarter the onion. Scrub and roughly chop the carrots and chop the celery. Add to the pan with the herbs.

3. Bring to the boil then cover, reduce heat and simmer for 1½ hours over a very low heat. Alternatively save fuel and time by cooking in a pressure cooker at 15 lb (6 kilos) pressure for 25 minutes.

4. When the stock is ready, strain and leave to cool. Skim off any fat before using. This stock freezes swell. Freeze in ice cubes and store in plastic bags, or freeze in plastic boxes.

Court Bouillon

Imperial (Metric)
1 carrot
1 onion
1 stick celery
1 bay leaf
3 parsley stalks
2 sprigs of thyme
Juice ½ lemon
¼ pint (150ml) dry white wine
¾ pint (450ml) cold water
6 black peppercorns

1. Peel and chop the carrot and onion. Chop the celery.

2. Put all the ingredients into a large saucepan, cover and bring to the boil. Reduce the heat and simmer for 20 minutes.

3. Leave to cool and strain before using. Court bouillon is used to poach fish.

White Sauce

(Makes ½ pint/300ml. Supplies 230 calories and 160mg sodium.)

Imperial (Metric)
½ oz (13g) unsalted butter or low-salt margarine
½ oz (13g) 85 per cent wholewheat flour
½ pint (300ml) skim milk

1. Melt the butter or margarine in a medium-sized pan over a low heat.

2. Add the flour. Stir in with a wooden spoon and cook gently for one minute. This mixture is known as a *roux*.

3. Gradually add the liquid, beating well and making sure the liquid is fully incorporated before adding any more. Continue to beat the sauce and allow it to come gently to the boil to let it thicken. The sauce is now ready for using.

Variations:
Make a thicker, coating sauce by doubling the amount of fat and flour. Make a binding, or *panada*, sauce by increasing the amount of fat and flour fourfold, i.e., 2 oz (50g) fat and 2 oz (50g) flour to ½ pint (300ml) liquid.

Low-sodium flavourings:
● Avoid adding salt; use a salt replacer or simply season to taste with lashings of freshly ground black pepper.
● Make a Béchamel sauce by simmering the milk for 10 minutes with a quarter onion, a bay leaf, 6 black peppercorns and a pinch of nutmeg before making the sauce.
● Substitute some of the milk for cider, white wine or vegetable stock.
● Flavour with 1 teaspoonful mustard.
● Add a handful of finely chopped parsley.
● Add 4 oz (100g) halved button mushrooms to the milk and simmer for 10 minutes, before straining and using the milk to make the sauce. Then return the mushrooms to the sauce when cooked.
● Lightly sauté 2 large onions in the fat, without browning, before making the sauce.

Rich Vegetable Sauce

Illustrated opposite page 65.

(Serves 4. Supplies 120 calories and 80mg sodium per portion.)

Imperial (Metric)
2 cloves garlic
8 oz (225g) onion
8 oz (225g) carrots
2 sticks celery
2 tablespoonsful olive oil
1 lb (450g) fresh tomatoes
4 tablespoonsful water
1 tablespoonful unsalted tomato purée
8 oz (225g) button mushrooms, wiped and sliced
1 green pepper, de-seeded and chopped
2 teaspoonsful oregano
Freshly ground black pepper

1. Crush the garlic. Finely chop the onion. Scrub and dice the carrots. Chop the celery. Cook all together in the oil for 5 minutes, without browning.

2. While cooking, skin the tomatoes by plunging each into a bowl of boiling water for 1 minute. Chop. Add to the pan with the water, tomato purée, mushrooms, pepper and oregano.

3. Bring to the boil, then cover and reduce the heat and simmer for 30 minutes. Season with freshly ground black pepper and serve.

Note: Serve this sauce either with cooked wholemeal spaghetti, cooked brown rice (to make a risotto), with aubergines, or to stuff peppers. Its uses are endless; it can also be frozen.

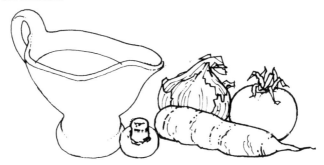

Tomato Sauce

(This quantity supplies 230 calories and 25mg sodium — 145mg if made with tinned tomatoes.)

Imperial (Metric)
4 oz (100g) onion
1 clove garlic
1 dessertspoonful oil
1 lb (450g) fresh tomatoes *or* 15 oz (425g) tinned
½ teaspoonful oregano *or* marjoram
1 green or red pepper (optional)
Freshly ground black pepper

1. Finely chop the onion and crush the garlic. Sauté together in the oil for 2 minutes.

2. If using fresh tomatoes, skin and roughly chop them and then add to the pan. Break up tinned tomatoes with the back of a spoon. Add herbs and de-seeded and finely chopped pepper if using.

3. Bring to the boil, then reduce the heat, cover and simmer for 20-25 minutes, stirring occasionally. The sauce should be quite thick and pulpy. Add freshly ground black pepper to taste.

Note: Serve with pasta, rice, as a topping for pizza, with courgettes, as an accompaniment to burgers or nut roasts, or as a base for chicken casserole (with a little extra water or stock).

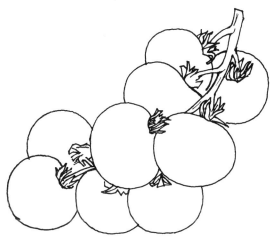

French Dressing

(Makes 4 tablespoonsful of dressing which supplies 550 calories and only traces of sodium.)

Basic recipe:

Imperial (Metric)
1 tablespoonful cider vinegar
3 tablespoonsful cold-pressed olive oil
Freshly ground black pepper

1. Place the vinegar, some black pepper and the oil in a clean screwtop jar and shake vigorously to blend together. Pour over salad and either chill and let flavours mingle, or serve at once depending on recipe.

Variations:
Cider vinegar has a valuable level of potassium but, if preferred, substitute another vinegar as appropriate. Avoid malt vinegar's rasping strength. Choose from white wine or red wine; raspberry; garlic; tarragon. Alternatively, substitute the juice of a lemon, or the juice of ½ orange. Cold-pressed olive oil is valued for its flavour but cold-pressed safflower or sunflower seed oils have higher levels of essential fatty acids and are best used for uncooked dishes.

Low-sodium optional extras:
For extra flavour use one of these, or a combination. Simply add with the oil and vinegar to the jar and shake well:

- ¼ teaspoonful ground cumin seeds.
- ¼ teaspoonful cayenne pepper or paprika.
- 1 teaspoonful caraway seeds.
- 1 teaspoonful mustard.
- 1 dessertspoonful salt-free tomato purée.
- 1 dessertspoonful chopped mint.
- 1 dessertspoonful tahini.
- 1 tablespoonful chopped chives.
- 1 tablespoonful chopped parsley.
- 1 tablespoonful chopped thyme.
- 1 clove garlic, crushed.
- 1 spring onion, finely chopped.
- 1 shallot, finely chopped.

Mayonnaise

(Makes ¼ pint/150ml. Each tablespoonful supplies about 300 calories and 5mg sodium.)

Mayonnaise should be made slowly, adding the oil to the yolks literally a drop at a time. Adding the oil too quickly will curdle the mayonnaise. If you have a blender make the mayonnaise in this; most models have a detachable centre to the lid; remove this and gradually add the oil through the hole. If you don't have a blender you will need a strong wrist to cope with the thorough beating needed to make a good mayonnaise.

Imperial (Metric)
2 egg yolks
Pinch of mustard powder
¼ pint (150ml) oil, ideally a blend of cold-pressed olive oil and either safflower or sunflower oil
½-1 teaspoonful cider vinegar
Freshly ground black pepper

1. Place the egg yolks in a blender goblet or in a mixing bowl. Add the mustard powder. Beat together.

2. Add a drop of oil and beat it in thoroughly. Continue to add the oil drop by drop, beating thoroughly in between. When all the oil has been added the mixture should be pale, thick and creamy. Then add the vinegar to taste, and season. If the mayonnaise separates then start again with another egg yolk in a clean bowl, adding the curdled mayonnaise a drop at a time. The mayonnaise will keep for a few days in the fridge. Use in salads which need a rich creamy dressing.

8.

BREADS AND BISCUITS

Sesame and Sunflower Rolls

Illustrated opposite page 80.

(Makes 10 rolls. Each supplies 150 calories and 4mg sodium.)

Imperial (Metric)
12 oz (325g) wholemeal flour
1 oz (25g) sesame seeds
1 oz (25g) sunflower seeds
1 oz (25g) low-sodium margarine
25mg vitamin C tablet, crushed
½ oz (13g) fresh yeast
1 teaspoonful clear honey
8 fl oz (240ml) tepid water
Milk to glaze

1. Place the flour and seeds in a mixing bowl and rub in the margarine.

2. Place the vitamin C tablet, honey and yeast in a jug and pour over the water. Stir well and then pour onto the flour mixture. Mix together to form a dough.

3. Turn out onto a lightly-floured surface and knead until smooth (about 5 minutes). Cover with an upturned bowl and leave to rest for 10 minutes.

4. While the dough is resting, lightly grease 2 baking sheets and heat the oven to 450°F/230°C (Gas Mark 8).

5. Divide the dough into 10 equal-sized pieces. Roll each into a ball, flatten slightly and place well apart on baking sheets.

6. Cover and leave to prove in a warm place until doubled in size. Glaze with milk and bake at the top of the oven for 15-20 minutes until golden-brown and the rolls sound hollow when tapped underneath.

Low-sodium Biscuits

(Makes 28. Each supplies 56 calories and 3mg sodium.)

Basic recipe:

Imperial (Metric)
6 oz (175g) wholemeal flour
1½ oz (38g) oatmeal
¼ teaspoonful nutmeg
¼ teaspoonful cinnamon
1 teaspoonful mixed spice
1½ oz (38g) low-sodium margarine
1½ oz (38g) unsalted butter
2 oz (50g) molasses sugar
1 egg
1 tablespoonful milk

1. Sieve the flour into a mixing bowl and add back the bran from the sieve. Mix in the oatmeal and spices.

2. Rub in the margarine and butter until the mixture resembles fine breadcrumbs. Stir in the sugar and mix in thoroughly.

3. Beat the egg with the milk and add just enough to the mixture to make a soft, but not sticky, dough. Reserve any extra egg and milk for glazing.

4. Roll out the dough on a lightly-floured surface to ¼-inch (5mm) thick and stamp out shapes with biscuit cutters. Transfer to lightly-greased baking trays.

5. Glaze with the remaining egg and milk and place in the centre of a pre-heated oven at 375°F/190°C (Gas Mark 5) for 15 minutes until golden-brown and just beginning to crisp up. Carefully lift straight away onto a wire cooling tray where they will crispen.

Variations:
● Substitute desiccated coconut for oatmeal.
● Add 1 teaspoonful ground ginger in place of the mixed spice.
● Add currants and grated rind of ½ lemon in place of oatmeal.

Oaty Bread

(Makes 1 small loaf which cuts into 10 slices, each supplying 90 calories and less than 2mg sodium.)

Imperial (Metric)
8 oz (225g) wholemeal flour
1 oz (25g) medium oatmeal
½ oz (13g) low-sodium margarine
½ oz (13g) fresh yeast
25mg vitamin C tablet
1 teaspoonful clear honey
¼ pint (150ml) tepid water
Milk to glaze

1. Place the flour in a bowl and stir in the oatmeal. Rub in the margarine.

2. Crumble the yeast tablet into the water and stir in the honey. When dissolved, pour onto the flour and stir in with the hands. Bring together to form a dough.

3. Turn onto a floured surface and knead until smooth (about 5 minutes). Cover with an upturned bowl and leave to rest for 10 minutes. Meanwhile grease a 1 lb (450g) loaf tin.

4. When the dough is rested, knead gently and then shape into an oblong, three times as long as the tin. Fold into three and, with the fold underneath, place in the tin. Cover and leave to double in size in a warm place.

5. Glaze with milk and bake in a pre-heated oven at 450°F/230°C (Gas Mark 8) for 25 minutes, until golden-brown. Tip the loaf out of tin and if it sounds hollow when tapped underneath, it is ready.

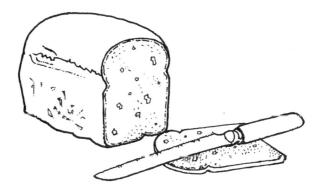

Savoury Seed Snaps

(Makes 24 biscuits. Each supplies 50 calories and 4mg sodium.)

Imperial (Metric)
8 oz (225g) wholemeal flour
2 oz (50g) low-sodium margarine
3 teaspoonsful sesame seeds
2 teaspoonsful poppy seeds
1 teaspoonful caraway seeds
½ teaspoonful cayenne pepper
1 free-range egg
Milk to mix

1. Light the oven and heat to 375°F/190°C (Gas Mark 5). Lightly grease 2 baking sheets.

2. Place the flour in a mixing bowl and rub the margarine into the flour until the mixture resembles fine breadcrumbs. Stir in the seeds and cayenne pepper.

3. Beat the egg and add to the flour mixture with just sufficient milk to mix to a soft dough. Knead lightly.

4. Roll out the dough on a lightly-floured surface to ¼-inch (5mm) thickness.

5. Cut out rounds using a plain edged cutter. Place each round on the prepared baking sheets.

6. Glaze with milk and bake in the centre of the oven for 15-20 minutes until golden and just crisp. Cool on wire trays.

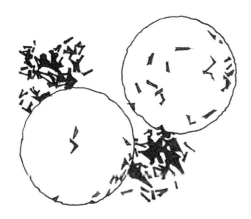

Herb Twists

Illustrated opposite.

(Makes 7. Each supplies 140 calories and 3mg sodium.)

Imperial (Metric)
8 oz (225g) wholemeal flour
1 oz (25g) low-sodium margarine
¼ pint (150ml) tepid water
25mg vitamin C tablet, crushed
½ oz (13g) fresh yeast
1 dessertspoonful oil
2 oz (50g) onion
2 cloves garlic
1 teaspoonful parsley, chopped
1 teaspoonful fresh sage, chopped
Beaten egg to glaze

1. Put the flour into a mixing bowl and rub the margarine in until the mixture resembles fine breadcrumbs.

2. Pour the tepid water onto the crushed vitamin C tablet, add the yeast and stir together well. Pour onto the flour and mix to a soft dough using hands.

3. Turn out onto a lightly-floured surface and knead until smooth (about 5 minutes). Cover with an upturned bowl and leave to rest for 10 minutes.

4. Heat the oven to 450°F/230°C (Gas Mark 8). Lightly grease a 7-inch (18cm) sandwich cake tin.

5. Finely chop the onion and crush the garlic. Sauté together in the oil for 2 minutes. Stir in the chopped herbs. Set aside.

6. Roll out dough to a rectangle about 8 × 12 inches (20 × 30cm). Spread the onion mixture over the dough and roll it up from the long side. Cut into 7 pieces and arrange, cut side up, in the tin.

7. Cover, and leave to double in size in a warm place (about 20 minutes). Glaze with beaten egg and bake at the top of the oven for 15-20 minutes until golden-brown.

Opposite: Savoury breads without a grain of salt. From the top: Sesame and Sunflower Rolls (page 76); Herb Twists (above); Walnut Bread (page 81).

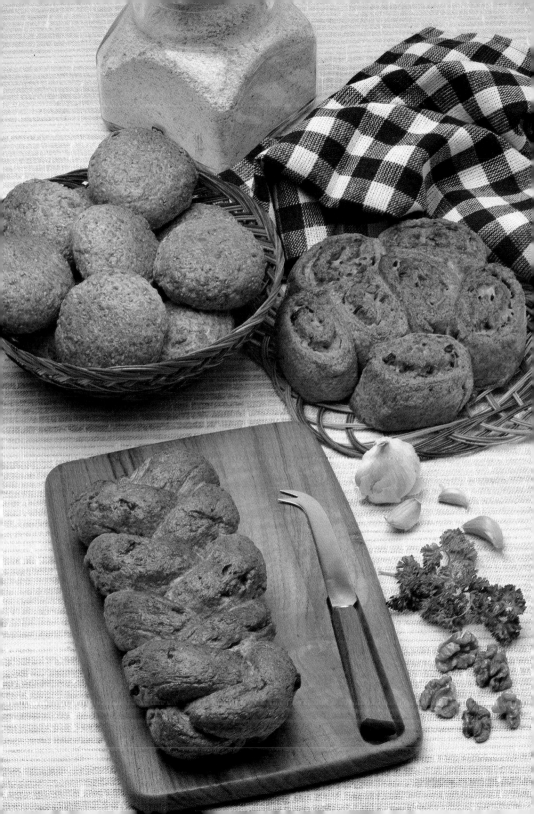

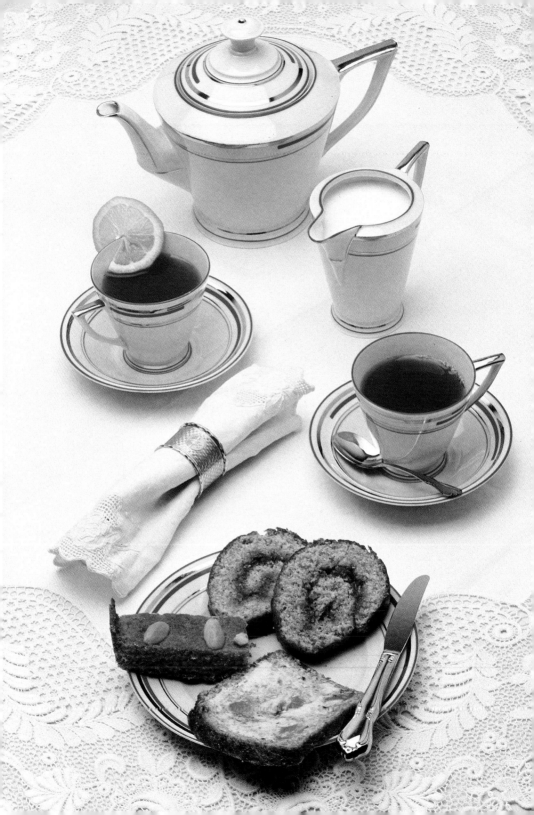

Walnut Bread

Illustrated opposite page 80.

(Cuts into 10 chunky slices. Each supplies 110 calories and 1mg sodium.)

Imperial (Metric)
8 oz (225g) wholemeal flour
2 oz (50g) walnuts, finely chopped
½ teaspoonful mustard powder
½ oz (13g) low-sodium margarine
¼ pint (150ml) tepid water
½ oz (13g) fresh yeast
25mg vitamin C tablet
1 teaspoonful clear honey
Milk to glaze

1. Place the flour, walnuts and mustard in a bowl. Rub in the margarine until mixture resembles fine breadcrumbs.

2. Pour tepid water onto yeast, crushed vitamin C tablet and honey. Stir well and pour onto flour mixture. Bring together with the hands to form a dough. Turn out onto a lightly-floured surface and knead until smooth (about 5 minutes). Cover with an upturned bowl and leave to rest for 10 minutes.

3. Lightly grease a baking sheet and heat the oven to 450°F/230°C (Gas Mark 8). Divide the rested dough into three. Gently roll each into a fine strip about 12 inches (30cm) long. Join the three together at one end by pressing together the ends of each strip. Plait loosely. Lift the plait onto the prepared baking sheet. Cover and leave in a warm place to double, about 25-30 minutes.

4. Glaze with a little milk. Bake in the centre of the oven for 20-25 minutes until golden-brown and when tapped underneath, sounds hollow. Serve either hot or cold.

Opposite: Teatime treats. Wholemeal Swiss-roll (page 87); Almond Finger (page 84); Apricot and Date Teabread (page 91).

Crunchy Wheat Bread

(Makes 1 loaf which cuts into 10 slices. 190 calories and 2mg sodium per slice.)

Imperial (Metric)
3 oz (75g) wholewheat grain
14 oz (400g) wholemeal flour
¼ pint (150ml) water
¼ pint (150ml) apple juice
¾ oz (20g) fresh yeast
25mg vitamin C tablet, crushed
1 dessertspoonful sunflower oil
Milk to glaze

1. Place the wheat grain in a pan of cold water. Bring to the boil, reduce the heat and simmer for 45-50 minutes until just soft. Drain.

2. Add the cooked wholewheat grain to the flour and mix together.

3. Mix the water with the apple juice and warm gently to tepid. Stir in the yeast and crushed vitamin C tablet.

4. Add the yeast liquid and the oil to the flour. Mix together with the hands forming a soft dough. Add a little extra flour if mixture is wet.

5. Turn out onto a lightly-floured surface and knead for 10 minutes until the dough is smooth. Cover and leave to rest for 10 minutes.

6. Heat the oven to 450°F/230°C (Gas Mark 8). Lightly grease a baking tray.

7. Divide the dough into three. Roll each out into a long strip, about 12-inches (30cm) long. Join the three together at one end and plait. Transfer to the prepared baking tray, cover and leave in a warm place to double (about 25-30 minutes).

8. Glaze with the milk, then bake at the top of the pre-heated oven for 20-25 minutes, until the loaf is golden-brown and, when tapped underneath, sounds hollow.

9.

CAKES AND DESSERTS

Sesame Flapjacks

Illustrated opposite page 49.

(Cuts into 15 pieces. Each supplies 230 calories and 10mg sodium.)

Imperial (Metric)
3 oz (75g) sesame seeds
6 oz (175g) low-sodium margarine
3 tablespoonsful clear honey
3 oz (75g) Demerara sugar
3 oz (75g) desiccated coconut
2 tablespoonsful sunflower seeds
6 oz (175g) rolled oats

1. Spread the sesame seeds over the base of a grill pan and put under a hot grill to toast lightly for a few minutes. The seeds should just colour; do not allow to burn.

2. Heat the oven to 325°F/170°C (Gas Mark 3). Lightly grease a Swiss-roll tin.

3. Place the margarine, honey and sugar in a large pan and heat gently until the margarine has melted.

4. Stir in the coconut, sunflower seeds, oats and sesame seeds. Mix together thoroughly. Remove from the heat and spread in the prepared baking tin, smoothing over top.

5. Bake in the centre of the oven for around 25 30 minutes until golden-brown. Mark into rough squares but leave in the tin to cool before cutting and removing.

Almond Fingers

Illustrated opposite page 81.

(Cuts into 10 slices. Each supplies 200 calories and 18mg sodium.)

Pastry:

Imperial (Metric)
4 oz (100g) wholemeal flour
2 oz (50g) low-sodium margarine or unsalted butter
1 egg yolk
Cold water to mix

Filling:

Imperial (Metric)
2 oz (50g) low-sodium margarine
2 oz (50g) light Muscovado sugar
1 egg yolk
3 oz (75g) ground almonds
2 oz (50g) 100 per cent wholemeal flour
1 oz (25g) desiccated coconut
2 tablespoonsful skim milk
2 egg whites
A few split almonds

1. Heat the oven to 350°F/180°C (Gas Mark 4). Rub the margarine or butter into the flour until the mixture resembles fine breadcrumbs.

2. Add the egg yolk and just sufficient cold water to mix to a soft, but not sticky, dough. Roll out and line a 7 or 8-inch (18 or 20cm) shallow square cake tin.

3. Cream the margarine with the sugar until light and fluffy. Beat in the egg yolk.

4. Sieve in the ground almonds and flour and add the coconut. Gently fold in with a metal spoon. Add the milk.

5. Stiffly whisk the egg whites and gently fold into the cake mixture. Pile into the pastry case and smooth over the top.

6. Sprinkle a few split almonds on top and bake for 20-25 minutes until well risen and the mixture springs back when touched with a fingertip.

Chelsea Buns

(Makes 8. Each supplies 180 calories and 13mg sodium.)

Imperial (Metric)
8 oz (225g) wholemeal flour
1 oz (25g) unsalted butter
3 fl oz (90ml) skim milk
2 fl oz (60ml) water
½ oz (13g) fresh yeast
25mg vitamin C tablet, crushed
1 dessertspoonful honey
1 egg yolk
½ oz (13g) unsalted butter, melted and cooled
2 oz (50g) dried apricots, chopped
2 oz (50g) sultanas
1 oz (25g) raw cane Demerara sugar
¼ teaspoonful cinnamon
Honey to glaze

1. Put the flour in a mixing bowl and rub in the butter.

2. Heat the milk and water until just warm and pour onto the yeast, vitamin C tablet and honey. Stir together well.

3. Pour the yeast liquid onto the flour mixture and add the egg yolk. Mix together thoroughly to form a soft dough, adding a little more flour if necessary.

4. Turn out onto a lightly-floured surface and knead until smooth (about 5 minutes). Cover with an upturned bowl and rest the dough for 10 minutes.

5. While the dough is resting, heat the oven to 450°F/230°C (Gas Mark 8) and lightly grease a 7-inch (18cm) sandwich tin.

6. Roll out dough to a rectangle 8 × 12-inches (20 × 30cm). Spread butter over the dough and sprinkle chopped fruit, sugar and cinnamon on top. Roll up from the longest side.

7. Cut into 8 pieces and arrange in a greased tin, cut side up, with one in the centre. Cover and leave to double in size in a warm place.

8. Bake in the centre of the oven for 15-20 minutes. Glaze with honey as soon as they come out of the oven and leave to cool in the tin.

Choux Pastry

(Supplies 710 calories and 142mg sodium.)

This quantity will make 10 eclairs or 14 profiteroles or alternatively form the base for a savoury gougère (just add ¼ teaspoonful mustard powder to the flour).

Imperial (Metric)
¼ pint (150ml) cold water
2 oz (50g) low-sodium margarine
2½ oz (63g) 85 per cent wholemeal flour, sieved
2 eggs, size 3

1. Place the water and margarine in a pan. Bring to the boil and immediately add all the flour.

2. Remove from the heat and beat the flour in thoroughly. Continue to beat until the mixture is smooth and glossy and leaves the sides of the pan.

3. Beat in one egg thoroughly until no traces remain. Add the second egg and again beat in well. The paste is now ready to use.

Fruit Profiteroles

(Makes 14. Each supplies 100 calories and 13mg sodium.)

Imperial (Metric)
1 quantity choux pastry (see above/opposite)
½ lb (225g) strawberries
¼ pint (150ml) double cream

1. Heat the oven to 425°F/220°C (Gas Mark 7). Lightly grease 2 baking sheets.

2. Place dessertspoonsful of the mixture well apart on the trays and bake, when oven is heated, at the top of the oven for 15 minutes. Turn down the temperature to 400°F/200°C (Gas Mark 6) to finish cooking.

3. Test after 10 minutes. Gently press the sides of the profiteroles; if they 'give' they are not ready. If firm they are done.

4. Remove them from the oven and gently slit the sides to let the steam out. Return to the oven for a final 5 minutes before cooling on a wire tray.

5. When the puffs are quite cool, whip the cream. Wash the strawberries and chop roughly. Fill each profiterole with some cream and strawberries.

Wholemeal Swiss-roll

Illustrated opposite page 81.

(Cuts into 8 slices. Each supplying 90 calories and 25mg sodium.)

Imperial (Metric)
3 eggs
3 oz (75g) clear honey
3 oz (75g) wholemeal flour
3 tablespoonsful 'no-added-sugar' raspberry jam

1. Grease a Swiss-roll tin and line with greaseproof paper.

2. Place the eggs with the honey in a large mixing bowl. Beat together, using an electric mixer, or with a hand whisk. If using the hand whisk, place the bowl above a pan of hot water to speed up the mixing. Whisk the mixture until it is pale, smooth and thick. Test by trailing the mixture into a letter W; if, when you make the last stroke, the first stroke is still visible, the mixture is ready.

3. Sieve the flour and dust some of the bran from the sieve in the lined tin. Sieve the flour again, this time into the egg and honey mixture. Fold it in very gently with a metal spoon. Pour the mixture into the tin. Bake in a pre-heated oven at 425°F/220°C (Gas Mark 7) for 10-12 minutes.

4. Have ready a sheet of greaseproof paper. When the Swiss-roll has shrunk away from the sides of the tin, and springs back when touched with a finger tip, it is ready.

5. Remove from the tin by turning it upside down over the sheet of paper. Place a wet tea towel on the base of the tin and leave it for a few seconds. Lift off the towel and then gently remove the tin. Peel off the paper and spread jam over the cake, trimming off ¼-inch (5mm) all round to neaten. Make a cut ½-inch (1cm) from edge nearest you. Roll the cake up around this and leave it to cool on a wire rack.

Almond Popovers

(Makes 9. Each supplies 180 calories and 8mg sodium.)

Imperial (Metric)
8 oz (225g) wholemeal flour
1 oz (25g) unsalted butter
3 fl oz (90ml) skim milk
2 fl oz (60ml) water
½ oz (13g) fresh yeast
25mg vitamin C tablet, crushed
1 dessertspoonful clear honey
1 egg yolk
4 oz (100g) raw cane sugar marzipan
1 oz (25g) split almonds
Egg white to glaze

1. Put the flour in mixing bowl and rub in the butter.

2. Heat the milk and water until just warm to the touch and pour onto the yeast, tablet and honey.

3. Pour the yeast liquid and egg yolk onto the flour and mix in thoroughly, drawing the mixture into a soft dough. Add a little extra flour if it is too sticky.

4. Turn out onto a lightly-floured surface and knead for 5 minutes until smooth. Cover with an upturned bowl and leave to rest for 10 minutes.

5. While dough is resting, heat the oven to 450°F/230°C (Gas Mark 8) and lightly grease 2 baking sheets. Knead the marzipan until pliable and divide into 9 equal pieces.

6. Roll dough out to a square 9-inch (23cm) and trim edges. Cut into 9 small squares. Roll each piece of marzipan into a ball and flatten slightly and place in the centre of each square.

7. Brush the edge of each square with a little egg white and fold each corner into the centre. Press the centre down well.

8. Place well apart on the greased baking sheets. Cover and leave to double in size in a warm place (about 20 minutes).

9. Glaze with egg white and bake in the centre of the oven for 10-15 minutes until well risen and golden-brown.

Carob Chip Cookies

(Makes 28. Each supplies 100 calories and 8mg sodium.)

Imperial (Metric)
4 oz (100g) low-salt soft vegetable margarine
6 tablespoonsful clear honey
1 egg
3 oz (75g) chopped almonds
¾ oz (18g) sunflower seeds, lightly toasted
¾ oz (18g) sesame seeds, lightly toasted
3 oz (75g) carob bar, finely chopped
8 oz (225g) wholemeal flour

1. Cream the margarine with the honey until fluffy. Beat in the egg.

2. Fold in with a metal spoon the chopped nuts, seeds and carob. Then sieve the flour into the bowl and add back the bran from the sieve. Fold in gently until thoroughly mixed.

3. Place small spoonsful on lightly greased baking trays and bake in a pre-heated oven at 375°F/190°C (Gas Mark 5) for 15 minutes until golden-brown. Transfer to a wire cooling tray to cool.

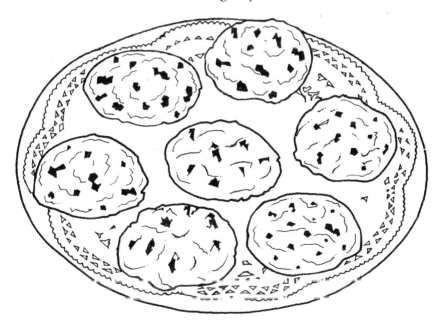

Date Slices

(Makes 16 slices. Each supplies 200 calories and 4mg sodium.)

Imperial (Metric)
12 oz (325g) dates
4 tablespoonsful water
Grated rind of ½ orange
2 tablespoonsful orange juice
8 oz (225g) wholemeal flour
4 oz (100g) rolled oats
3 oz (75g) Demerara sugar
5 oz (150g) low-salt margarine

1. Roughly chop the dates and place in a pan with the water, orange rind and juice. Cook gently for 5 minutes, until dates are soft and pulpy. Allow to cool while preparing the topping.

2. Lightly grease a Swiss-roll tin, 8 × 10 inches (20 × 30cm). Light the oven 375°F/190°C (Gas Mark 5).

3. In a large mixing bowl, mix together the flour, oats and sugar. Melt the margarine over a low heat and stir into the flour mixture thoroughly.

4. Spread half the mixture in the base of the tin. Spread the date mixture on top and finally lightly cover with the remaining flour mixture.

5. Bake in the oven for 25-30 minutes, until golden-brown. Mark into squares and allow to cool in the tin.

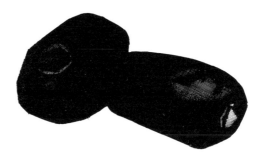

Apricot and Date Teabread

Illustrated opposite page 81.

(Makes 1 loaf which will cut into 10 slices. Each slice supplies 115 calories and 72mg sodium.)

Imperial (Metric)
½ teaspoonful cinnamon
Pinch of nutmeg
8 oz (225g) wholemeal flour
1 oz (25g) low-sodium margarine
¼ pint (150ml) tepid water
1 dessertspoonful clear honey
½ oz (13g) fresh yeast
25mg vitamin C tablet
2 oz (50g) dried apricots
2 oz (50g) dates
Milk to glaze

1. Lightly grease a 1 lb (450g) loaf tin. Stir the spices into the flour and rub in the margarine.

2. Pour the water onto the honey, yeast and crushed vitamin C tablet. Stir well and, when the yeast has dissolved, pour onto the flour mixture. Use your hands to bring the mixture together to form a soft dough.

3. Turn out onto a well-floured surface and knead for 5 minutes until quite smooth. Cover with a bowl and leave to rest for 10 minutes.

4. While the dough is resting light the oven 450°F/230°C (Gas Mark 8). Put the apricots into a small bowl and cover with boiling water. Leave to soak for 10 minutes. Chop the dates and the soaked apricots.

5. Flatten the dough and place the chopped fruit in the centre. Knead in the fruit thoroughly. Press the dough gently into an oblong three times as wide as the tin. Fold into three and place in the tin. Cover and leave to prove in a warm place for about 25-30 minutes. The loaf should double in size and the dough should spring back when touched with the fingertip.

6. Glaze with milk and bake for 20 minutes. Remove from the tin and lightly tap the base. The loaf should sound hollow. Cool on a wire tray.

Apple Crumble

(Serves 5. Supplies 280 calories and 8mg sodium per portion.)

Imperial (Metric)
4½ oz (113g) wholemeal flour
2 oz (50g) rolled oats
2 oz (50g) soft vegetable margarine
2 cloves
½ teaspoonful cinnamon
2 oz (50g) Demerara sugar
1½ lb (675g) Bramley cooking apples
Juice of 1 lemon
Cold water
1 tablespoonful clear honey

1. Place the flour and oats in a bowl. Rub in the margarine finely. Stir in the spices and sugar. Heat the oven to 400°F/200°C (Gas Mark 6).

2. Peel, core and slice the apples. Cover with apple juice and some cold water as you slice them, to stop them from browning.

3. When all the apples have been sliced, arrange the slices in the base of an ovenproof dish and add the honey and 1 tablespoonful of the water and lemon juice mixture.

4. Cover with the crumble mixture and bake in the centre of the oven for 20-25 minutes until the topping is brown and the apples are just soft.

Variations:
Substitute other fruits for the apples — plums, rhubarb, blackberries and apricots are all suitable.

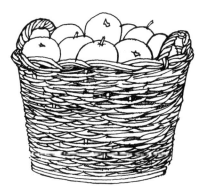

Fresh Fruit Salad

(Serves 5. Supplies 125 calories and 4mg sodium per portion.)

Imperial (Metric)
3 tablespoonsful cold water
1 teaspoonful clear honey
2 oranges
1 small bunch black grapes
1 small bunch white grapes
8 oz (225g) plums *or* strawberries
2 peaches
2 red skinned eating apples
2 eating pears
Juice of 2 lemons
1 banana

1. Put the water and honey in a small pan and heat until the honey has dissolved. Set aside to cool.

2. Peel the oranges and cut into segments, discarding the pith. Wash and halve the grapes, removing the seeds.

3. Wash the plums, if using, halve and remove their stones. Wash and hull the strawberries, if used.

4. Peel the peaches and chop the flesh.

5. Core and finely slice the apples, mixing with lemon juice to prevent browning. Peel, core and chop the pears and lastly slice the banana.

6. Either arrange the fruit in layers in a large glass serving bowl or mix together. Pour on the syrup.

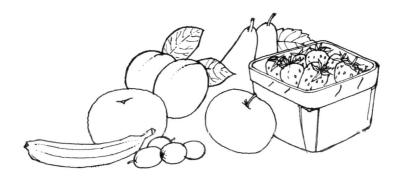

Fruit Sorbet

(Serves 4. Supplies 88 calories and 30mg sodium per portion.)

Imperial (Metric)
2 oz (50g) fructose
¼ pint (150ml) cold water
1 lb (450g) soft fruit — strawberries, raspberries, kiwifruit or melon
2 egg whites

1. Put the fructose and water in a small pan and heat gently until the fructose has dissolved. Boil for 1 minute and remove from heat. Leave to cool.

2. Prepare the fruit of your choice, peeling kiwifruit or melon, if used. Place in a liquidizer with the syrup and blend until smooth. Sieve to remove any pips (not necessary if using melon or strawberries).

3. Transfer the mixture to a shallow polythene container and freeze for 3 to 4 hours until just mushy.

4. Beat with a fork to break up any ice crystals. Stiffly whisk the egg whites and gently fold in with a metal spoon.

5. Return to the freezer and freeze until firm — this takes about 3 hours.

6. When ready to use, take out of freezer about 10 minutes before serving to soften. Then scoop out and serve in individual glasses.

INDEX

Addison's disease, 9
aldosterone, 9
Almond and Mushroom Bake, 49
    Fingers, 84
    Popovers, 88
Apple Crumble, 92
Apricot and Date Teabread, 91
Aubergine Curried with Spinach
    and Potato, 62

Bean Salad, Mixed, 59
Biscuits, Low-sodium, 77
blood pressure, high, 8, 9
bread, 17
    and biscuits, 76-82
breakfasts, 22-25
butter, unsalted, 18

Cabbage Sauté, 61
cakes and desserts, 83-94
Carob Chip Cookies, 89
Cauliflower and Cashew Rice,
    Curried, 52
    Soup, 28
Celery, Apple and Walnut Starter,
    31
Chelsea Buns, 85
Chicken Dopiaza, 45
    Risotto, Summer, 58
    Stock, 70
Chilli Beans, 44
chloride, 7
Choux Pastry, 86
Cod and Mushroom Pie, 41
Coley and Courgette Braise, 43
Coleslaw, 66

Courgette and Cauliflower Pasta
    Salad, 67
    and Tarragon Soup, 26
Courgettes, Stuffed, 32
Court Bouillon, 70
Croissants, Wholemeal, 22
Crudités, 33
Crunch, Breakfast, 25
Cucumber and Grape Salad, 66

Date Slices, 90
Dolmades, 36

eggs, 19
E numbers, 12

fats, polyunsaturated, 18
fish, 18
flour, wholemeal, 18
foods, plant protein, 19
French Beans, Spicy, 63
    Dressing, 74
fruit, 19
Fruit Salad, Fresh, 93
    Sorbet, 94

Green Salad, Tossed, 60
Guacamole, 34

Haricot Goulash, 51
Health Education Council, 7
heart disease, 8, 18
herbs, 16
    and spices, 16
Herb Twists, 80
Hummus, 33
hypertension, 8, 9

Khichhari, 47
kidney failure, 8, 9

Lamb Kebabs, 57
Lamb's Liver Casserole, 50
Leek Soufflé Quiche, 48

Macaroni Medley, 42
Mackerel Parcels, 35
MacGregor, Graham, 8
main courses, 35-58
margarines, low-salt, 18
Marrow Rings, Stuffed, 39
Mayonnaise, 75
meat, 18
Minestrone, 29
Muesli, 23
Mulligatawny Soup, 27
Mushroom and Okra Rice, 68
Mushroom Quiche, 46
Mushroom Salad, Tangy, 65
Mushrooms à la Grecque, 30

National Advisory Committee on
    Nutrition Education (NACNE),
    7, 9

Oaty Bread, 78

Pizza, 38
potassium, 7, 9, 16, 19
Potato with Carrot, Spicy, 61
Potato Salad, 65
protein, 18
Prunes, Cinnamon, 23

Ratatouille, 62
Rice Ring, Chilled, 64

salt intake, 7-9

low-sodium, 15
    substitutes, 16
Scotch Eggs, 37
Seed Snaps, Savoury, 79
Sesame and Sunflower Rolls, 76
Sesame Flapjacks, 83
sodium, 7, 11, 19
    additives, 11, 12, 17
    flavourings, 17
    foods, 13-14
soups and starters, 26-34
Spinach, Pancakes Stuffed with,
    56
stocks, sauces and dressings,
    69-75
Summer Pie, 54
Sweetcorn Chowder, 28
Swede Purée, 60
Swiss-roll, Wholemeal, 87

Tomato Sauce, 73
Tomatoes, Stuffed, 30

U.S. Senate Select-Committee on
    Nutrition and Human Needs,
    7

Vegetable Pasties, 40
    Sauce, Rich, 72
    stock, 69
vegetables, 19
    and salads, 59-68
vitamins:
    B, 19
    C, 19

Walnut Bread, 81
    Patties, 53
Wheat Bread, Crunchy, 82
White Sauce, 71

Yogurt, Natural, 24